I0663814

DR. LYNCH'S HOLISTIC SELF-HEALTH PROGRAM

DR. LYNCH'S HOLISTIC SELF-HEALTH PROGRAM

Three Months to Total Well-Being

JAMES P. B. LYNCH, D.C.
WITH ANITA WEIL BELL

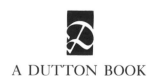

A DUTTON BOOK

A NOTE TO THE READER:

The ideas, procedures, and suggestions contained in this book are not intended as a substitute for consulting with your physician. All matters regarding your health require medical supervision.

DUTTON
Published by the Penguin Group
Penguin Books USA Inc., 375 Hudson Street,
New York, New York 10014, U.S.A.
Penguin Books Ltd, 27 Wrights Lane,
London W8 5TZ, England
Penguin Books Australia Ltd, Ringwood,
Victoria, Australia
Penguin Books Canada Ltd, 10 Alcorn Avenue,
Toronto, Ontario, Canada M4V 3B2
Penguin Books (N.Z.) Ltd, 182–190 Wairau Road,
Auckland 10, New Zealand

Penguin Books Ltd, Registered Offices:
Harmondsworth, Middlesex, England

First published by Dutton, an imprint of Dutton Signet, a division
of Penguin Books USA Inc.
Distributed in Canada by McClelland & Stewart Inc.

First Printing, March, 1994
10 9 8 7 6 5 4 3 2 1

Copyright © James P. B. Lynch and Anita Weil Bell, 1994
All rights reserved

 REGISTERED TRADEMARK—MARCA REGISTRADA

LIBRARY OF CONGRESS CATALOGING-IN-PUBLICATION DATA:
Lynch, James P. B.
  [Holistic self-health program]
  Dr. Lynch's holistic self-health program: three months to total well-being / James P. B.
Lynch with Anita Weil Bell.
    p.   cm.
  Includes bibliographical references.
  ISBN 0-525-93760-9
  1. Holistic medicine.   2. Self-care, Health.   3. Health.
I. Bell, Anita Weil.   II. Title.   III. Title: Holistic self-health program.
R733.L95   1994
613—dc20   93–33558
                                                                                CIP

Printed in the United States of America
Set in Century Book
Designed by Leonard Telesca

Without limiting the rights under copyright reserved above, no part of this publication may be reproduced, stored in or introduced into a retrieval system, or transmitted, in any form, or by any means (electronic, mechanical, photocopying, recording, or otherwise), without the prior written permission of both the copyright owner and the above publisher of this book.

Contents

PART THREE
SELF-HEALTH RESOURCES

Acknowledgments

This book would not have been possible without the driving force that motivated me to become a holistic doctor: the premature deaths of my beloved parents, James and Johanna Lynch. After experiencing the health care system, and how it contributed to their deaths, I was determined to help change health care for the better.

I would also like to acknowledge the loving support of my family and my wife, Ann.

Appreciation to Dr. William Holub and the other physicians and healers who taught me to rely on the natural healing power of the body; and to the late Dr. Robert Mendelsohn for his honest, inspiring work. Many thanks to the patients of the Holistic Health Force, from whom I have learned a great deal.

Thanks to Anita Bell, for her hard work and dedication. Much gratitude to our literary agent, Faith Hamlin, for her enthusiasm; and our editor, Carole DeSanti, for her guidance and expertise.

Anita Bell thanks her parents, Shirley and Gilbert Weil, for their love, interest, and support. And a heart full of gratitude to her husband, Jonathan Bell, for his positive attitude, creative spirit, and unconditional love.

Finally, we wish to acknowledge the inner healing force that is the natural order of the Universe and the power of love.

Introduction

Would you like to meet the greatest healer in the world? Look in the mirror. *You* are your own best doctor.

Every person possesses an innate healing force. This book will teach you how to use this powerful healing force to love and nurture yourself into optimal health.

Good health is your natural birthright; it's not a commodity you need to pay for with frequent visits to overpriced M.D.'s. The power to create good health and enjoy life to the fullest lies within *you*. Your own knowledge, faith, love, and actions are far more powerful and effective than any pill or scientific "advance."

The purpose of the Three-Month Holistic Self-Health Program is self-empowerment: to help you learn to help yourself. As a holistic doctor I consider myself first and foremost a teacher. I am a partner in healing with my patients, and now I hope to be your partner.

Since you're reading this book, you're probably interested in alternatives to traditional medical care. Perhaps, like millions of other people, you're dissatisfied with the inflated costs and market mentality of orthodox medicine. You may be sick and tired of doctors who patronize you and don't take the time to consider your unique needs. Perhaps you've suffered side effects from prescription drugs or have endured unnecessary or unsuccessful surgery.

Your motivation to explore holistic health might have been prompted by a serious illness, a nagging complaint, or concern about your future. Whatever your current state of mind and body, you will be healthier and stronger when you finish the Natural Self-Health Program. You'll take greater responsibility for your own health and enjoy the fruits of independence. You'll be part of the holistic health revolution.

The holistic health revolution is as necessary as our American Revolution of 1776. The medical establishment has evolved into an empire, primarily concerned with its own power and riches rather than the well-being of its "subjects." Of course, there are many sincere and dedicated physicians, and there's a place for the techniques of conventional medicine. But there is also an urgent need for a massive overhaul of the system. It's crucial that we begin to focus on prevention and natural remedies instead of drugs and surgery.

The holistic health revolution involves a growing number of individuals who make health care choices based on solid, scientifically tested knowledge. They visit alternative health care professionals such as nutritionists, chiropractors, massage therapists, herbalists, homeopaths, acupuncturists, and others. They adopt more healthful diets and utilize supplements and herbs. *Instead of waiting for symptoms to happen, they take steps to balance their bodies and minds so that ailments are less likely to occur.*

The term "holistic" stems from "wholistic." It means consideration of the whole person: body, mind, and spirit. It's interesting that the word "health" finds its roots in the Anglo-Saxon word *hal,* or "whole." Yet the term "medical care" derives from "medicine," something given as a remedy for disease. In truth, medical care is generally *disease* care rather than *health* care.

Consider *Webster's New World Dictionary*'s first definition of health: "physical *and* mental well-being." If you think about it, you'll realize that a system that recognizes the integral connection between the body and mind is truly *health* care, while a system that concentrates solely on the physical is *disease* care.

The basic difference between the medical approach and the holistic approach is that medicine treats the *symptom* while holistic health care treats the *whole person* and the *root* of the symptom. For example, if you have migraine headaches, instead of prescribing a drug that temporarily blocks the pain, a holistic practitioner will investigate dietary, emotional, and physical factors until the cause of the pain is discovered and addressed.

Medical care often involves smothering the symptom with drugs or, when the situation worsens, surgically altering the body. Holistic practitioners *respect* the symptom. We search for the root cause and try to correct the imbalance without insulting your body any further. It sounds like simple common sense, doesn't it? Yet this basic approach is unknown to modern medicine.

Medical science tends to make disease sound too complicated for laypeople to understand. Yet the truth about disease is actually simple.

The basis of all disease is the same: toxemia, or poisoning, and/or imbalance of the body. The body is in a state of health when all the organs and systems are in balance and harmony and free of toxins. And this can be achieved only when you take responsibility and proactive steps to maintain your own well-being. Holistic healers can help, but no one can do it for you. Ultimately your health is in your own hands.

I first became aware of the powerful connection between the mind and body when I studied martial arts as a teenager. By the time I gained my black belt, I knew on a deep level that the mental, spiritual, and physical components of a human being were interconnected and interdependent. I sought a way to integrate this knowledge with my goal to become a doctor.

My desire to become a doctor had been triggered when my mother died of heart disease and my father died of cancer, both at relatively young ages. It was clear their deaths were brought on by poor dietary habits, stress, and exposure to toxins. I wanted to help other people avoid our family's tragedy by becoming a doctor who teaches people how to take care of themselves.

Modern chiropractic training, with its emphasis on healing the whole person and teaching prevention, was the path I chose. I was also attracted to the intensive study of nutrition included in the curriculum of chiropractic college.

Once I established my own practice, I was determined to help patients learn how to stay balanced and well instead of merely providing them with temporary relief. However, I found that most people could understand the principles of holistic health intellectually but were unable to apply these ideas to their own lives. They were well intentioned but found it difficult to nurture all aspects of their body/mind without a structure.

To help my patients apply the principles of holistic health and prevention more effectively, I developed the Holistic Triangle. This approach has proved to be extremely successful. During my fifteen years of practice, hundreds of people have not only overcome persistent ailments but learned to live healthier lives using this model.

The Holistic Triangle is a teaching tool, a healing tool, and a means of helping you direct your thoughts and actions. The Holistic Triangle puts your health in your own hands. There are three sides to the Holistic Triangle: the mental/spiritual base, the physical side, and the chemical side.

In this book we will explore in depth what each side of the Triangle represents. You'll learn about the strengths and weaknesses of each side of your Triangle and how they influence your life. You'll discover how the three sides of your Triangle—mental/spiritual, physical, and chemical—interact.

Here are some basic examples: What you eat (the chemical side) affects your mood (the mental/spiritual side) and your energy level (the physical side). Exercising (the physical side) affects your metabolism (the chemical side) and makes you more positive and alert (the mental/spiritual side).

Most important, knowledge and self-love (the mental/spiritual side) give you the inner strength to eliminate toxins (the chemical side) and stay with an exercise regimen (the physical side). The mental/spiritual base *supports* the other sides of the Triangle and enables you to take healthy action.

The foundation of health is nourishing your mental/spiritual side with love. *Love is the most powerful healing force.* Unconditional love for yourself is the basis of health and the most essential nutrient.

This is not narcissism but the true self-love that enables you to do right by yourself and by others. Loving yourself actually reduces selfish behavior by enhancing your ability to love others and have a positive influence on the world.

You may be worried that you don't love yourself enough and don't have the mental/spiritual strength to take healthy action. I ask you from my heart: Have an open mind and give yourself a chance. *You can learn to love yourself.* There are practices and ways of thinking that can help you relax into the self-love and good health that are your natural state.

Then you can continue on to the next steps of nourishment. You can detoxify your body and adopt a wholesome, individualized diet with appropriate supplements. You can nourish your physical side with oxygen by committing yourself to an exercise program specially designed for your abilities and needs. You can learn which holistic practitioners complement your self-care. It's all part of the Three-Month Holistic Self-Health Program.

This program is a step-by-step plan to improve every aspect of your well-being by nourishing your Holistic Triangle. It's a user-friendly program designed for real people, not saints. Everyone has lapses, and part of the program is learning to forgive yourself and get back on the right track.

The program begins with Self-Health Evaluation questionnaires to help you learn about the state of your Holistic Triangle. You'll gain motivation to start the program and the commitment to stay with it.

The first month of the program focuses on developing your mental/spiritual side with practices and self-education. Once your mental/spiritual side is reinforced, you'll be ready to build and limber up your body by starting an exercise program.

The second month emphasizes detoxification and replacing

low-nutrient foods with fresh, energy-giving foods. You'll eliminate toxins, develop healthier eating habits, and enjoy a variety of nature's food. You'll benefit from raw-juice fasting—that is, refraining from all food and drink except raw juices—during this period, as you continue your exercise and mental/spiritual practices.

The goal of the final month of the program is to reach a higher level of physical fitness by revving up your exercise program. You'll probably find yourself feeling and looking leaner, younger, and stronger this month. And by the end of the program you'll be remarkably rejuvenated and energized.

This may sound overly optimistic, but it's based on many years of experience. In my practice, which is called the Holistic Health Force, patients are guided through their own Self-Health Programs. My primary goal is to help my patients become self-sufficient so they don't need me anymore!

My patients' programs include office treatments, but these are often secondary in importance. It's what people do when they are on their own that counts most. The results of this approach are astonishing and inspiring. People not only overcome health problems but transform their lives in many ways.

I don't mean to give the impression that it will be a breeze for you to attain excellent health and create a better life for yourself. In fact, I can promise the opposite: the Holistic Self-Health Program is not a magical panacea; it's hard work. Accomplishment is directly proportional to the amount of attention you put into your Triangle. However, it's enjoyable work. You'll have fun during the process and see a lot of improvement along the way. The more steps you take to love yourself to health, the more satisfaction you'll feel, which in turn will increase your self-esteem. Instead of the infamous downward spiral, the program will take you on an upward trajectory.

As you shift to a holistic lifestyle, you'll be enlivened by your increased knowledge, your spirituality, your exercise activities, and your nourishing diet. You won't live forever, but you'll probably live longer, and the quality of your life will be enhanced. You'll be a positive influence on those around you and on society, instead of being a victim of civilization.

The major diseases in our society—heart disease, cancer, diabetes, obesity, and addictions—all are natural consequences of an artificial environment that we call civilization. We're not winning the war against these killers because our resources are being misdirected.

Nourishing your Holistic Triangle will help you live in better harmony with the forces of the natural world and activate your innate healing force. It will enable you to create a sanctuary for yourself in the midst of the modern world. It will give you the energy and love you need to live a joyous, healthy life.

PART ONE

YOUR HOLISTIC TRIANGLE

CHAPTER 1

Getting to Know
Your Holistic Triangle

Is there a nagging health problem you want to eliminate? Are there aches or pains you wish to erase? Perhaps you want to have more energy and a higher level of fitness.

Do you need to relax and let go of tension? Do you want to be more optimistic and positive? Do you want to free yourself from guilt and fear? Would you like to develop your spiritual side?

All these changes, and more, are possible. The innate healing force is within you, and the power to change is in your hands. You can begin the process by learning about your Holistic Triangle, which you form with your hands.

Holistic Triangle

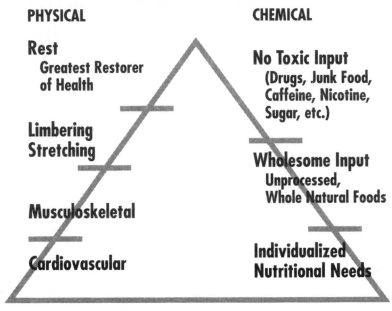

PHYSICAL

Rest
Greatest Restorer
of Health

**Limbering
Stretching**

Musculoskeletal

Cardiovascular

CHEMICAL

No Toxic Input
(Drugs, Junk Food,
Caffeine, Nicotine,
Sugar, etc.)

Wholesome Input
Unprocessed,
Whole Natural Foods

**Individualized
Nutritional Needs**

Mental + Spiritual
Worst Mental Enemies: Fear and Guilt
Worst Spiritual Enemies: Rejection and Lack of Faith

HOW THE HOLISTIC TRIANGLE WAS BORN

In the early years of my practice I often discovered that patients wanted to consider their health in a holistic way, but they found it confusing or overwhelming to accomplish this without a road map. So I began to imagine a symbol that would bring holistic principles to life and enable them to be practically applied. It had to be a symbol that connected as well as delineated the components of holistic health.

The classical holistic trilogy or triangle is: Mind-Body-Spirit. Although this is a beautiful and profound trilogy, I found many patients couldn't relate to it, and it wasn't always workable in a practical sense. Many people thought the Mind-Body-Spirit trilogy sounded too mystical and far-out. Others thought having "Body" in one massive category was confusing.

My biggest problem with Mind-Body-Spirit trilogy was the separation of mind and spirit. In my experience it's *putting together* mind and spirit that works. Knowledge and faith need to support each other to instill the will to action. Therefore, the mental/spiritual side became the base of the Holistic Triangle I developed. I also found that defining the physical and chemical components of the body helped people identify their weaknesses and strengths and learn to nourish every aspect.

To form the Triangle, use your thumbs and forefingers. Stretch out your thumbs horizontally, one thumb resting on top of the other. Lift up your forefingers diagonally so your fingertips touch at the apex of the Triangle.

Your thumbs represent your mental/spiritual side, which is the foundation of health. The mental and spiritual elements, like your thumbs, overlap and support each other. The right side of the Triangle, formed by your right forefinger, represents the chemical side. The left side of the Triangle represents your physical side.

You can remember these sides easily with this association: The physical side is on the left because your heart is on the left, and your heart is the major cardiovascular organ. The right denotes the chemical side since the liver, the primary detoxifying organ, is on the right side.

Although the mental/spiritual, chemical, and physical sides each have unique qualities, they are interdependent and interactive. The three sides work together to create your total health picture. Nourishing one side of your Triangle supports and strengthens the other sides.

The Holistic Triangle is a symbol of your health. The Triangle is a teaching tool, a learning device, and, I hope, a source of inspiration. This may sound dramatic, but symbols can have tremendous power if you believe in what they represent. The more you learn and think about your Triangle, the more it will influence your decisions and your life.

In the following chapters, you'll learn many practical ways to nourish your Holistic Triangle. But first let's get acquainted with each side.

YOUR MENTAL/SPIRITUAL SIDE

Do you know the ABC's of self-health? Attitude, Belief, and Consistency. The mental/spiritual side of your Triangle is the support system for the ABC's and the foundation of well-being.

The mental side is about understanding the basic truths about health. The concepts that follow are some of the major principles:

- Good health is not merely the absence of symptoms; it is the state in which all your organs and systems are in balance and harmony.
- Diseases or symptoms are natural communications from your body and it's vital to discover their message. Smothering symptoms with drugs deprives you of valuable information about yourself.
- Lasting good health comes from discerning and correcting the root causes of symptoms and taking steps to prevent recurrence.
- Good health comes from healthful practices.

The two worst enemies on the mental side are fear and guilt. Conventional medical practice can instill fear when it assumes a superior, patronizing stance. And patients who don't swallow their doctors' prescriptions are sometimes made to feel guilty.

Holistic practitioners strive to eliminate the fear that springs from the unknown and promote understanding, awareness, and responsibility. You might think that being responsible for your own health will make you feel guiltier than ever. But the truly holistic approach is to understand how your actions and thoughts may be affecting your health and to be motivated to change because you love yourself, not because you feel guilty.

The mental side of the Triangle involves *knowing* what makes you truly well. But in order to put what you know into practice, you need to develop the spiritual aspect: faith in the innate healing force with which you were born.

Perhaps you'd like to believe in your self-healing force, but you're skeptical. Since most of us were trained to trust outside authority and not ourselves when it comes to our health, it's no wonder you have doubts. Don't worry if you don't start off with faith in your natural healing power; you can cultivate it.

There are three main ways to gain faith:

1. The intellectual approach: reading about holistic princi- ples, case histories, and research studies.
2. Practices: prayer, meditation, Healing Moments, relaxation, and visualization. These practices help you *feel* the truth on a deep level.
3. Personal experience: perhaps the most powerful way to cultivate faith in natural healing. When you go through the Natural Self-Health Program, you'll see for yourself the power of your inner healing force.

The fundamental nourishment on the spiritual side is love. I can't repeat this too often: *Love is the most powerful healing force in the Universe.* When you love yourself, you treat yourself with care and respect. You take action to activate your self- healing and preventive measures to maintain well-being. The foundation of good health and happiness is unconditional, nonjudgmental self-love.

Think for a moment about whether or not you give yourself un- conditional love. Do you treat your body with consideration and respect? Do you accept yourself or berate yourself for shortcom- ings? Do you take time out for the nourishment and relaxation you deserve? Do you encourage and forgive yourself? Do you treat yourself as well as you treat your best friend?

If the honest answer to some of these questions is no, don't feel defeated or inadequate. Most of us have negative program- ming we need to overcome. You don't have to remain stuck in any mental state. You can lose emotional baggage just as you can lose weight. You can transform the way you think just as you can change the contours of your body. You can actually *learn to love yourself.*

Of course, all human beings are fallible, and there will be times when you don't love yourself. But instead of continuing on a downward spiral, you can learn to nourish your Triangle and get back on the upward track of self-love. In this book you'll learn practices and ways of adjusting your thinking that can help you achieve self-forgiveness, overcome the effect of negative parenting, and relax into the nourishment of self-love.

Mental/spiritual strength can make all the difference in the healing process. Two patients, John and Bill, each came to my office complaining of lower back pain. John was thirty-five years old, about forty pounds overweight, strong but heavy. Bill was thirty-two years old, about twenty-five pounds overweight, and out of condition. John had played football in high school and then steadily acquired his beer belly throughout college and his working years. Bill had been naturally slim until after college, when he started eating out a lot and gaining weight. Both men had sedentary jobs and no regular exercise regimens.

John and Bill had each been to their medical doctors and had gone through courses of painkillers and rest that afforded only temporary relief. When they went back to work and off the drugs, the pain returned.

Their examinations yielded similar findings: Both men had discogenic sciatica, commonly known as slipped disk. In the office I gave John and Bill similar treatments: spinal adjustments, traction, and diathermy (electrical induction of heat into the tissues below the skin). I also explained that they needed to lose weight, take early-morning baths, and commit themselves to following a gentle exercise program to strengthen their spines and decompress their vertebrae. Their participation was the most vital aspect of their treatment programs.

John was enthusiastic about the prospect of curing himself of back pain. He liked the idea of being in control instead of helpless under a doctor's care. His attitude was: "I *will* do it; I *can* do it." John worked out at the gym, did relaxation exercises, modified his diet, and lost weight. Within two months he no longer needed my professional services, except for a seasonal tune-up. Over the next six months he kept losing weight until he was back down to what he called "fighting trim."

Bill, on the other hand, kept coming back with excuses. He

was too rushed to bathe in the morning. He didn't have time to join a health club and go swimming. He didn't want to give up the lavish late-night dinners he enjoyed. His attitude was: "I would, *but*—" and "Can't *you* do something?"

Bill wanted to be free of pain, but he wanted someone else to do it for him. Predictably the office treatments weren't enough to cure his back problem without his own efforts. Bill became disenchanted with the holistic approach and decided to go to a "real expert." He ended up having spinal surgery: a discectomy and laminectomy (removal of the disk and spinal fusion).

The surgery gave Bill only temporary relief from pain, and he wound up with failed back syndrome, a medical term for people who have chronic back pain even after spinal surgery. (It's interesting that it's called failed back syndrome instead of failed back surgery.)

Two men with similar histories and diagnoses, yet one becomes pain-free, trim, and fit; the other ends up with chronic pain. The moral of this true story is obvious: It's imperative to have a sturdy mental/spiritual foundation, to have faith in the natural healing process, and to take action to help it along.

YOUR CHEMICAL SIDE

The right side of your Holistic Triangle represents the chemical component of health. This involves everything you take into your body: food, drink, drugs, and supplements.

Nowadays there is a great deal of concern about pollution on the planet. But many of us don't pay enough attention to how we pollute our own bodies. And our bodies are one environment over which we as individuals do have control.

By detoxifying your body through dietary changes and fasting, you can create an optimally healthy "in-vironment." Not only will you have immediate benefits, but you'll also be less likely to develop a serious disease. The American Heart Association, American Diabetes Association, and National Cancer Institute, among others, have recognized the link between diet and the major killers. And natural healers have known this for centuries.

The number one tool on the chemical side of the Triangle is detoxification, eliminating toxins and cleansing your body. The Top Ten Toxins you'll be working to eliminate are sugar, white flour and refined carbohydrates, dairy products, red meat, food additives (including extra salt), caffeine, nicotine, alcohol, drugs, and environmental toxins.

Please don't let the list of toxins stop you in your tracks. This will be a gradual process, and you'll be gaining far more than you give up. You'll be adding to your diet a variety of fruits, vegetables, and grains, natural foods that are energizing as well as delicious.

Yes, it can be difficult to give up your favorite poisons, but it's not as hard as you might think. This is where the interaction of the three sides of the Triangle comes into play. Empowering your mental/spiritual side will give you the information and inspiration you need for the task of detoxification.

Giving up toxins doesn't mean you'll end up feeling deprived. Sure, it's hard to break bad habits, but there are many delicious, nutritious alternatives you can enjoy. These "Garden of Eden" foods come from the original source of energy: the sun. High-energy natural foods can help you feel better and younger now than you did at twenty (especially if you were partying and eating junk food at that age). You'll also learn to nourish your holistic Triangle through appropriate vitamin, mineral, and herbal supplementation.

YOUR PHYSICAL SIDE

The physical side of your Triangle encompasses your genetic inheritance and structure and your level of fitness. This is the side of the Triangle where we deal with what we've been given and what we've done with it.

Since we can't change our genetic legacies, the focus here is on how we can improve our bodies through physical nourishment. The primary form of physical nourishment is exercise. A holistic exercise program consists of aerobic (cardiovascular) exercise, musculoskeletal development exercises, and stretching. The holistic approach is to concentrate on proper breathing, technique, and form instead of on competition.

Secondary forms of physical nourishment are those that are provided by practitioners, such as chiropractic care, massage, and other natural physical therapies. As part of developing your physical side, it's likely you'll want to have periodic treatments from a professional. An overview of the different options on page 109 can help you pick the practitioner who suits your needs.

This is not to say you should give up your medical doctor altogether. There is certainly a place for medical expertise, and physicians can be incomparable in cases of serious trauma. But you can also benefit from the different services of holistic or complementary practitioners. The idea is to learn about alternatives and make informed choices instead of remaining locked into traditional care.

INTERACTION

Each side of your Holistic Triangle influences and interacts with the other two sides. A simple example of this process is exercise. Exercise is the number one nutrient on the physical side, but it also has an immediate affect on the mental/spiritual side. Endorphins, chemicals naturally produced by the body during exercise, evoke "runner's high," a sense of euphoria. Even nonaerobic exercise can lift your mood, enhance concentration, and instill a feeling of confidence. On the chemical side, exercise can lower tension and raise awareness. Then you'll be inclined to make healthy food choices and be less likely to overeat.

You've probably experienced how exercise affects all three sides of the Triangle, and you've undoubtedly felt the opposite results after overeating. A heavy meal can cause you to feel sluggish and unable to do anything more taxing than watch TV or take a siesta. That's the chemical side influencing the physical and mental sides of your Triangle.

Take a minute to think of some examples of this interaction from your own life. If you've experienced constipation, consider not only your diet but also your mental state. Were you tense, preoccupied, or under pressure? What about the physical side? Were you exercising regularly?

If you have frequent neck or back pain ask yourself: Do I hold emotional stress (the mental/spiritual side) in my body? Does my diet leave me feeling lethargic, so I can't uphold good posture (the chemical and the physical sides)? Do I care for myself enough to devote time and money to seeking out natural treatment (the mental/spiritual and physical sides)?

Once you see how it works, you can apply the "Three Sides of the Triangle" test to any health problem you may have. It's amazing the solutions you'll discover when you begin to think this way.

When you're investigating a health issue, remember to look at the *whole* picture. This includes your environment, your relationships, and your job.

Jill, a patient who had chronic neck and shoulder pain, worked in cytology, examining Pap smears and identifying cancers. Regardless of what treatment I could offer, there was no way she could spend all day peering down a microscope and not have this recurring pain.

Another contributing factor was that she felt her work was depressing and stressful, a "downer." Jill realized that her Holistic Self-Health Program had to include a change of career. Once she had identified this, she took necessary steps to obtain credentials to be a nutritionist. Now Jill enjoys looking up at people instead of down at cells. And she no longer has chronic neck pain.

You probably won't have to do anything as drastic as change your career. But you do need to consider every element of your life when you plan to improve your health. Everything you do, everyone with whom you're involved are part of the whole picture of wellness. Creating total well-being can at times involve changing your lifestyle as well as your diet.

MOTIVATION

It can be difficult to accept that good health requires effort and persistence especially since our society encourages instant gratification and the quick fix.

When Tony, a middle-aged factory worker, came into my office complaining of back pain, he asked me to "crack" his vertebra into place. He wanted a quick adjustment that would give him relief without any effort on his part. He didn't want to hear that he would have to stop sleeping on his stomach and cut down on drinking to shed the extra pounds that were stressing his back. When he learned that to alleviate his back ailment permanently, he needed to get involved in a comprehensive program, Tony cut out and went elsewhere to look for his "crack."

Well, Tony was back four months later. Although he had found a chiropractor who was willing to give him adjustments without an accompanying program, his back pain kept recurring. Finally, he was fed up to the point where he was willing to do some work on his own.

In the long run *quick fixes don't work*. The painkiller that is potent today may no longer be effective in a few months or may induce harmful side effects. Even a natural treatment won't provide permanent relief unless the root cause of the problem is addressed and corrected. And then it will be necessary for you to take steps to prevent the ailment from recurring. Good health is a gift that only you can give yourself.

Why bother? First of all, so you can eliminate your symptoms and enjoy a pain-free, high-energy life right now. Secondly, so you can live a longer life, with better health in your later years. Changing to a more healthful lifestyle will give you great rewards *now* and may save your life *later*. A holistic lifestyle means living for the moment *and* the future.

Sometimes I need to play the devil's advocate and warn patients about ailments that might develop in the future to motivate them to take preventive steps in the present.

Kimberly, a twenty-five-year-old dancer, came to see me about an ankle problem. She went through our usual office procedure, which begins with filling out a comprehensive wellness assessment. This includes a clinical history and family health information; questions on diet, exercise, and daily habits; and mental/spiritual/emotional components. (You'll be taking similar Self-Health Evaluations as part of the program.)

After I reviewed Kimberly's questionnaire, we sat down for a consultation. I explained the concept of the Holistic Triangle and how a "do-it-yourself" Holistic Health Program would result in overall health enhancement as well as relief of her symptom.

Kimberly was enthusiastic when I outlined the physical treatments and therapeutic exercises that would alleviate her ankle pain. But she was defensive when I pointed out that her wellness assessment indicated she was addicted to sugar. Kimberly protested that she was slender and energetic enough to teach modern dance, so why shouldn't she enjoy her chocolate treats?

Then I explained to her the connection between sugar addiction, hypoglycemia, and diabetes (see details on page 50). Since Kimberly's grandmother had died of diabetes, this information struck home. Kimberly decided to kick her candy habit. Two months later she reported that she was less moody and had even more energy than before. More important, she was no longer setting the stage for adult-onset diabetes.

When you think about your health and the state of your Triangle, consider the future. If you're a twenty-six-year-old mother who doesn't have time for therapeutic exercise, you may feel okay now, but will you develop osteoarthritis in twenty years? If you're a husky young man with an active job, you may be able to wolf down steaks without gaining weight, but are you setting yourself up for heart disease? You need to consider the whole picture: your history, the way you feel now, and the consequences your present lifestyle will have in the future.

GETTING YOUNGER

By working on the three sides of your Triangle, you may be able to slow down the aging process. You may be able to look and feel younger than you did five or even ten years ago. If this sounds farfetched, consider the following:

Research at the U.S. Department of Agriculture's Human Nutrition Research Center on Aging (HNRCA) at Tufts University has shown that people can control the ten major factors associated with aging. These "biomarkers" are: lean body mass, strength, basal metabolic rate, body fat percentage, aerobic capacity, blood pressure, insulin sensitivity, cholesterol/HDL ratio, bone density, and body temperature regulation.

Through diet, exercise, and relaxation techniques, you can in effect lower your physiological age. You can also reduce or eliminate many of the symptoms associated with aging.

Frank, a sixty-five-year-old retired businessman, was slowed down by arthritis. His symptoms were early-morning stiffness, pain that worsened when he used his joints, and restricted mobility. His doctor had prescribed aspirin and NSAIDs (nonsteroidal anti-inflammatory drugs), but these medications gave him gastrointestinal distress and ulcers. Instead of enjoying the retirement for which he and his wife had saved and planned, Frank felt old and miserable.

On the mental/spiritual side Frank needed to rethink his belief that nothing could help his arthritis. Reading several books on natural approaches to alleviating arthritis helped convince him there was hope.

The chemical side of his program involved reducing his intake of acidic foods and meat and eating more fruits. He also started taking appropriate supplements and drinking raw juices. Frank was skeptical about these dietary efforts, but his wife insisted he give them a try.

To nourish the physical side of his Triangle, Frank started a daily exercise program of gentle isometrics and swimming. His secondary treatment included diathermy and physical therapy.

After three months Frank no longer had early-morning stiffness and pain. He had greater energy and flexibility and had lost ten pounds. He reported that he felt younger than he had for fifteen years.

As long as he doesn't overdo it, Frank rarely has pain from the arthritis or gastrointestinal distress. He and his wife frequently go on Elderhostel trips and occasionally even go out dancing.

You're never too old, or too young, to feel younger. Many people have reported that by getting rid of toxins, increasing exercise, and improving their mental/spiritual aspect, they feel better at forty than they did at thirty.

The yogis have a saying, "You're only as old as your spine." I'd like to amend that to: "You're only as old as your Triangle."

SELF-EMPOWERMENT

Traditional medical care often creates a feeling of helplessness. My goal as a holistic doctor is to help patients activate their own natural healing ability. Self-empowerment is the basis of the holistic approach.

Self-empowerment can have dramatic results. Jan, a British woman in her early twenties, suffered from ankylosing spondyitis, a disease that is thought to be genetic and causes calcification of the spine. Jan had been told by medical doctors there was nothing they could do about her condition, and she was receiving disability payments. She lived like an invalid, with low self-esteem and frequent depression.

When Jan came to the Holistic Health Force, we did a blood work-up and took X rays that showed she had a mild case of ankylosing spondyitis. I told her there was no reason she couldn't live an active, fulfilled life.

Her program consisted of a more healthful diet and supplements, chiropractic work to take the biomechanical stress off her spine, and a gentle exercise regimen. Except for biweekly office treatments for three months, the bulk of the program involved self-help steps.

For the first time Jan believed she had some control over her condition. Her outlook changed tremendously. The listless, self-effacing person who had first come to see me was transformed into a vibrant young woman brimming with plans and enthusiasm. She enrolled in college and started dating for the first time.

Even more than any of the physical improvements gained by her program, it was thinking about her health in a new way that changed Jan's life.

CREATE YOUR OWN GARDEN OF EDEN

Our "civilization" is rife with uncivilized behavior, hardship, and stress. One key to well-being is to create a sanctuary for yourself and simulate paradise as much as possible.

On the mental/spiritual side, creating a sanctuary means feeling close to the Higher Force, however you experience God, the Universe, or your personal spirituality. It's letting go of guilt and returning to a state of peace and love without fear.

On the chemical side of the Triangle, a return to the Garden of Eden means eating the foods that were available in paradise: fresh fruits and vegetables, whole grains, seeds, and nuts.

Imagine how free and physical you might be in a "Garden of Eden" in your imagination. You might swim, run, walk, climb, stretch, dance, and play. On the physical side we want to aim for bodies that are as flexible and strong as the days before "civilization" glued us to our seats.

Let's take a practical look at how a few people create their own sanctuaries:

As soon as Leslie gets home from work, before she listens to her answering machine or looks at her mail, she goes into her bedroom and turns on a blue light. She finds this light soothing and comforting. Then she changes into loose clothes, stretches out on a mat, and does an hour of relaxation and yoga exercises. This switches her out of her workday worry mode for the rest of her evening.

Jeffrey used to slam the snooze button on his alarm clock every weekday morning. Then he'd be running late and would have to rush out of the house and grab a Danish and coffee on the train to work. By 11:00 A.M. he was usually in a mental slump and had frequent tension headaches. Now he gets up a little earlier and spends a relaxing, contemplative time in the bath, then has a nourishing breakfast. He wakes up looking forward to his morning ritual, instead of being instantly thrust into rush-hour anxiety.

Karen could afford either a one-week winter vacation or a year-long membership to a health club. She chose the health club and decided to make it into a minivacation two or three times a week. At her club she pretends she's at a luxurious spa and pushes herself through a vigorous workout. Then she goes to the sauna, where she concentrates on relaxing every inch of her body. After a shower she massages herself with herbal body lotion. She feels rejuvenated several times a week instead of once a year.

A NEW WAY TO START YOUR DAY

How do you start your average day? Does an alarm clock jolt you out of bed, straight to the kitchen, where a cup of coffee gives you another jump start? Do you rush through your shower and grab a quick bite? Do you already feel exhausted and harried by the time you start work?

Try a different routine that can change your entire day. First, switch to a clock radio that awakens you to pleasant music. Then, when you first wake up, begin by stretching a little in bed and taking a few deep breaths.

Think about what you can do that day to nourish your Holistic Triangle. On the mental/spiritual side perhaps you'll plan to stop by a bookstore and pick out a self-help book. Or you'll be sure to sit down for a stretching session when you get home from work (see page 215). On the chemical side you might want to plan a fresh salad you'll have for lunch or a visit to a health food store. On the physical side you might determine to push a little harder in your exercise class and then reward yourself with a foot massage.

After you get out of bed, I recommend doing the Bathing Ritual (detailed on page 219). Then you can enjoy a nutritious breakfast and take your supplements.

You'll be amazed at the difference this new morning routine makes for the rest of your day. You'll be taking control of your environment instead of allowing it to control you. Your energy and concentration levels will be higher; your body will be more relaxed, and your outlook will be brighter.

Sounds great, you may be thinking, but you don't have time for all that on a weekday morning. Perhaps you barely make it to work on time even when you rush.

If this is your situation, you need to establish new priorities. If you want to change your life and enjoy a balanced body/mind, you need to prioritize time to work on your Triangle.

Setting new priorities may mean you swim after work instead of joining your friends at Happy Hour. You could meditate instead of going to the mall. You think about what will enable you to feel good later, instead of what is escapist fun at the moment. You give up a few "junk food" activities to make time to nurture your Triangle.

Visualize yourself in glowing good health, filled with love and optimism. Then remind yourself that this picture is obtainable. It's a matter of choice.

Start with one little choice. Start by changing your routine in one small way. When the snack cart rolls around, eschew the doughnuts and go to the rest room for a private stretching session instead, or go outside for a ten-minute walk. Read up on a new subject that interests you instead of succumbing to TV. Make a tofu stir-fry instead of a meat dinner for your family. Spend thirty dollars on a shiatsu massage instead of a fattening restaurant dinner. On Sunday afternoon take a long, brisk walk instead of loafing and watching a ball game. The possibilities for nourishing your Triangle are limitless, and the choice is yours.

Changing your routine, making a different and healthier choice in one little way, will get you started. You'll gain faith in your ability to change. You'll realize you can choose love instead of fear. You can choose natural remedies instead of drugs. You're gaining inner strength and faith. Your Holistic Triangle is already getting stronger.

CHAPTER 2

The Mental/Spiritual Side of Your Holistic Triangle

When you form the Holistic Triangle with your hands, your thumbs overlap to form the mental/spiritual base of your Triangle. This symbolizes that your mental and spiritual strengths support each other to create the basis of good health. You need a fortified mental/spiritual base for wellness just as a building needs a sturdy and balanced foundation.

NOURISHING YOUR MIND

The mental aspect of this side of the Triangle means knowing the truth about health and disease. First, you may need to free your mind of the clutter of propaganda and misinformation about medicine and disease you've probably accumulated over the years. Then you can look at health from a fresh perspective.

The mental foundation of the Triangle includes understanding the basic truths about health. To review these concepts:

- Love is the most powerful healing force. When we love ourselves, we take action to get and keep ourselves well.
- Good health comes from healthful practices.
- Good health is a gift only you can give yourself. You must take responsibility for your own health if you want long-term wellness.
- Good health is the state in which all the organs and systems are in balance and harmony and free of toxins.
- The body has its own innate wisdom and inner healing force. The most effective way to get well and stay well is to learn to stimulate and utilize your natural healing force.
- The basis of disease is toxemia and imbalance of the body, not germs.
- You must listen to your symptoms, not smother them with painkillers, if you want to achieve lasting wellness. Listening to your symptoms means focusing on how the quality of your life affects the quality of your health.

Once you have established these principles in your mind, you can expand your knowledge. It's useful to have basic books in your home library on vitamins, herbs, natural healing arts, meditation and visualization, massage, and alternative health care. Books on these topics can be found in well-stocked mainstream bookstores, New Age bookstores, and some health food stores, as well as libraries.

A list of recommended readings is on page 229. You may want to use this list as a starting point if you find the choices in the bookstores and libraries overwhelming. But you can also browse and make your own selections, or ask friends about books they've found helpful.

Instead of reading primarily about subjects with which you're already familiar, try to expand your knowledge base by delving into areas in which your Triangle is weak. For example, if you already practice visualization, instead of reading another book on this subject, perhaps you could benefit more from reading a book on vitamins or acupressure. Spiritual reading is nourishing on a deep level, but you also need practical, hands-on books that teach you how to boost your health.

If you have a specific ailment, see if you can find a book with an all-natural, drug-free approach toward healing this problem. Many books on nutrition, supplementation, and herbology also have special sections on various maladies.

You'll find yourself turning to your favorite books time and time again once you become your own best doctor. Although you'll still need professional guidance, research can give you insights that expensive visits to an M.D. might fail to provide. A few examples:

Eddie, in his mid-forties, had endured a painful problem with hemorrhoids for more than fifteen years. He went through tubes and tubes of hemorrhoid medications, which did nothing more than temporarily relieve symptoms. When his doctor finally recommended surgery, Eddie was nearly desperate enough to try it. But a friend lent him a book on natural remedies for common ailments, and Eddie read about rutin, a bioflavonoid supplement available in health food stores. He found that taking rutin regularly, along with increasing his intake of water and fiber foods, cured his hemorrhoids within a few weeks.

Pilar had suffered from severe headaches for five years. She had been to several experts who prescribed costly drugs, such as Demerol, which caused disturbing side effects: extreme fatigue, drowsiness, and slurred speech. When Pilar became pregnant, she realized that she would have to survive for nine months without any drugs for migraine relief. She picked up a book on natural headache relief and learned acupressure massage and relaxation techniques she could do herself. These methods afforded such relief she decided to stay off the headache pills even after her child was born.

Patricia had been vulnerable to cold sores, or herpes simplex, on her lips since she was a teenager. Sometimes these sores lingered for weeks, causing her embarrassment and discomfort. After Patricia became interested in holistic health, she read that lysine, an amino acid, was useful in treating cold sores. The next time this problem occurred, she used an ointment containing lysine on her lips and also took lysine capsules. This time the cold sores didn't spread, and after three days they had completely dried up.

People have been able to help themselves overcome a host of physical ailments simply by reading books and magazine articles. Another bonus of becoming informed is that you can share your knowledge and help your friends and family. You may learn information that saves a loved one from needless pain and illness.

Audio- and videotapes are another way to nourish your mental side. Audiotapes can be particularly effective in guiding you through meditations and spiritual work, while videotapes can lead you through yoga classes and other exercise sessions.

Seminars, workshops, and courses are another excellent way to strengthen your mental base. In some communities chiropractors, nutritionists, and other holistic healers give complimentary lectures and programs. There's also a wide variety of courses, workshops, lectures, and seminars available for a fee, which can range from five dollars for a brief lecture to thousands for an extensive program.

The amount of time and money you should spend on a course depends on your financial resources and your degree of interest. Don't be talked into investing a great deal if you're not sure you're interested or you can't afford it. Attend an introductory lecture or demonstration, or read something the teacher has written before you sign up. It's certainly worth spending money on your mental side, but you don't want to end up feeling cheated. Courses can change people's lives, but they can also be disappointing. You need to be sure the person leading the program is truly an expert and a compassionate teacher.

Embark on the course with an open mind and a positive attitude, but don't have unrealistic expectations. Remember, you can't put your health and happiness in anyone else's hands, including holistic teachers or practitioners. It's not just what you learn and what you know; it's what you *practice* with consistency that creates change.

This brings us to the most important truth about nourishing the mental side of your Triangle: *It's what you do with your knowledge that really counts.* You can read books on meditation from here to nirvana, but if you don't practice, you won't gain peace of mind. You can stuff yourself with information about nutrition, but if you keep eating the wrong foods, it won't help. Don't let reading about holistic health become mere escapism. It won't work unless you practice what you learn.

How do you gain the discipline, motivation, and tenacity to carry through on what you have learned? By strengthening the spiritual aspect of the mental/spiritual side of your Holistic Triangle. It's putting together the mental and the spiritual that provides the alchemical magic. Love and faith are the fuel that turn knowledge into action.

There are many ways to gain faith in the natural healing force. You can read about cases and research studies. You can talk to holistic professionals and their patients about their experiences. You can look at nature's incredible way of restoring balance and the spontaneous healing in all forms of life.

You can also gain faith by thinking about all the times you've experienced your own natural healing power. Remember all the colds, flus, and other illnesses from which you have recovered? You might have taken medicine to ease the symptoms, but it was your innate healing force that made you well. Think of all the aches and pains that vanished after a good night's sleep. Consider the way your skin heals after a scrape or bruise. The regenerative healing force is within you, and all around you, every day.

Faith in the innate healing force and knowledge about natural healing techniques will give you a good start on strengthening your mental/spiritual side. But in order to realize your full potential, you need the self-love to turn right thinking into action.

LOVE IS THE MOST POWERFUL HEALING FORCE

Now that you're a critical thinker about health, you may ask, *Why* is love the most powerful healing force? How does love create good health?

The answer is simple. If you love and accept yourself, you will nourish yourself with healthy actions. When you love yourself, you *care*, and you believe that you're worth taking care of. It's not enough to *know* what is right. You need the self-love, discipline, and faith to *act* on what you know.

When we talk about love's creating health, we are not talking about romantic love or even familial love. Love from other people is precious beyond words, as everyone knows. And receiving love has been found to help people have longer and healthier lives. Everyone acknowledges the importance of love between people. But we must also realize the tremendous power of self-love.

This kind of self-love is not narcissism. Self-love does not mean thinking that the world revolves around you or that you're the best tennis player, the wittiest wordsmith, or the most attractive person in your crowd. In fact, this type of egotism reflects insecurity, rather than genuine self-love.

Genuine self-love means self-acceptance. It means working to accept and love yourself more fully every moment, every day, in every way, despite any qualities you may view as shortcomings. Self-love means loving yourself just the way you are, without criticism, without comparison, without conditions or requirements. It means loving and accepting yourself with a round belly or wrinkles around your eyes or a low-paying job.

At first it might sound as if this degree of self-acceptance will stand in the way of self-improvement. You may wonder, If I accept myself totally as I am, why bother to change? But you'll find that self-love actually motivates change and removes blocks. When you stop criticizing and fighting yourself, you free up a great deal of energy that you can redirect more productively. Fear will no longer hold you back. You can break through the denial or fear that keeps you from making changes. You'll have more confidence that you're capable of change.

When you love yourself, you respect your body and treat it with more care. You take the time and effort to nourish yourself with healthy food and exercise. You feel closer to your spiritual center. You have a greater capacity to love others and attract fulfilling relationships. You forgive and let go of anger and guilt, which can undermine your health. Your life is uplifted with optimism and hope.

The Holistic Triangle is designed to help you nourish all aspects of your self. And the most important nutrient of all, the nutrient that is the catalyst for all self-nourishment, is love.

All infants are born with an incredible capacity for love. However, our upbringings and life experiences can either reinforce and cultivate this self-love or suppress it. Parents who did not have nurturing upbringings themselves are sometimes unable to love their children unconditionally. Many people have to deal with childhood legacies of verbal, physical or sexual abuse, neglect, or abandonment. There are also the more subtle underminings of critical, perfectionistic, withholding, or smothering parents.

The cycle continues when children grow up to re-create these unloving scenarios with spouses and within themselves. And so the legacy of low self-esteem and destructive behavior is carried on from generation to generation. Later life experiences, both societal and personal, can also have a devastating effect on innate self-love.

This is, of course, a simplification of a complex subject. Family dynamics and self-esteem are multifaceted issues and are explored in many excellent books. Reading on these topics can help you gain tremendous insight into your mental/spiritual side and can also be very comforting.

SEEKING PROFESSIONAL HELP

Psychotherapy is an option to consider if you feel you need professional guidance to break through the barriers to self-love. There's a great deal you can do on your own to build self-esteem and learn to love yourself more. But depending on your life experience, you may want help. No one can make the decision for you. You need to think through your situation quietly and look within your own heart.

If you decide to seek professional help, look for a therapist with whom you feel relaxed and trusting. Choose one who is a loving, positive influence. Therapists can be professional and appropriate and still exude feelings of care and love for their patients.

If your gut instinct tells you the therapist is the wrong person for you, trust it. It's not enough for the professional to have a wall of certificates. You must feel a genuine connection with the person.

You might seek a mental health professional who is in tune with the basic principles of holistic health and knowledgeable about the influence of diet and exercise on moods. It's helpful if he or she is supportive of self-help techniques as a complement to your work together.

Unless you have a serious, biochemically based mental disorder, such as severe depression, manic depression, or schizophrenia, be wary of mental health professionals who are quick to prescribe psychoactive drugs. This is an area in which you need to proceed with great care and become as informed as possible. The long-term effect of psychoactive drugs as well as the short-term results should be carefully considered. The ultimate goal should be strengthening your Holistic Triangle so that medication is no longer needed.

If you cannot afford private counseling but need help in dealing with serious issues, there are several options. One is to visit a community mental health center, which may have lower or sliding scale fees. You can also look into counseling with a religious leader.

Joining a self-help or peer support group is another option. Al-Anon is a wonderful program for adult children of alcoholics, and there are also support groups for incest survivors, substance abusers, and people with behavioral addictions. Even if the group you find in your area doesn't focus on your specific experience or issue, the love and support from peers can be valuable.

Whatever barriers and traumas you need to overcome, remember, *the capacity for self-love is always within all of us.* In fact, those who have to overcome hardships and work harder at self-love often end up to be the most loving, spiritual people. Negative experiences can ultimately turn out to be life-enhancing because they compel people to gain insight, forgive, and grow stronger.

All of us, even those with very loving and supportive parents, can benefit by making a conscious decision to love ourselves more. We will explore several techniques that can help us do so later in this chapter. But first let's review some simple ways to build self-love that are so obvious you may be missing them.

HEALTHY, LOVING LIVING

Sheila hated herself for being overweight and overstressed. She couldn't break out of the tension/food binge/remorse cycle that started when she was in college, more than twenty years ago.

When Sheila came for treatment, she had a number of related complaints: gastrointestinal distress, constipation, and lower back pain. I explained to Sheila that she needed much more than chiropractic treatment. She needed to start treating herself in a loving way by taking healthy action.

Sheila read a number of books on deep relaxation and positive thinking, as well as on diet and nutrition. She began to recognize stress buildup and turn to relaxation techniques, meditation, and exercise as stress busters.

It was difficult for her to break her old pattern of filling up with junk food to deal with her stress and unhappiness. There were days when she managed to lie down and practice deep breathing or go for a quick walk to relieve her anxiety, but there were also times when she lost herself in eating binges. But now she was conscious of why she was binging and aware that she had the power to break the pattern. I kept reminding her that even when she binged, she could still come out ahead if she refused to wallow in self-hatred afterward.

After several weeks of struggling through her Holistic Self-Health Program, Sheila found her efforts had a "reverse domino" effect. The more she nourished her Triangle, the more she loved herself and the better she was able to cope with stress. Her digestive problems were reduced as she stayed with a healthier diet and practiced relaxation techniques. Over a period of three months she gradually lost weight and gained self-confidence. Even when the old self-loathing and negative thinking crept up on her, Sheila tried to react by *doing* something positive: by nourishing one of the sides of her Triangle.

Taking healthy action is a primary way to love yourself and raise your self-esteem. When you feel stuck in your mind or your habits, *do something nourishing*. Put on a favorite record from your teenage years, and dance around your room like crazy. Make yourself a lavish fruit salad. Lie down on your floor and practice deep breathing. Do something that will sustain your Triangle, not deplete it. You can choose whatever it is, but do it *consciously*.

Act, don't react. Quick fixes—routines that you know are bad habits—leave you feeling worse. Stuffing yourself with ice cream provides only a brief rush of childish solace, but in the long run it's going to make you feel worse. A shopping binge may be a temporary distraction, but it may leave you feeling guilty and broke. Think about not only how your action causes you to feel while you're doing it but how you'll feel later.

Remember, truly nourishing actions have only positive side effects.

The habit of blaming others for your state of mind or body is a trap, one from which you must free yourself. Again, the theme of simultaneous freedom and responsibility is paramount. You are responsible for your mental health, as well as your physical well-being, and you need to show love for yourself by taking action.

One of my most inspiring patients is Jane, a thirty-one-year-old woman who developed multiple sclerosis when she was twenty-five. She had difficulty walking, and the left side of her body was spastic. She also had general muscle weakness, vertigo, and bladder problems. Her medical doctors had offered no substantial intervention and said all she could do was wait and see how her disease progressed.

Jane used what little energy she had to take care of her husband, whom she had married at a young age, and her ten-year-old son. She continued doing everything for others and nothing for herself, as she had done all her adult life.

When Jane became a holistic patient, she realized that she had to devote more energy and time to herself. Her Holistic Self-Health Program of supplementation, dietary changes, physical therapy, exercise, and mental/spiritual work would take up part of her day. To create time for the program, it was necessary to assert herself with her husband and ask him to share some of the household work.

Confronting her husband with the need for change and relinquishing some of her caregiving responsibilities was the most difficult step for Jane. But she realized she had to devote more love on and attention to herself to fight her disease, and she took action.

Jane was seriously motivated and went into her Self-Health Program with a lot of determination. Since she was shifting from an unhealthy lifestyle, the results of her program were dramatic. Within three months her multiple sclerosis had started to go into remission. Her friends noticed that her gait had improved and her energy level was much higher. She reported that her husband was now glad he had taken over some of her chores so that she could have time to help herself.

After years of feeling that she was helpless against her disease, Jane was deeply affected by the positive changes that came about through her program. She was committed to continuing the diet, supplementation, therapeutic exercises, and other elements. When I last saw her, about two years after she had started the program, her MS was still in remission and her energy level was high.

LOVING OTHERS

The more love you give, the more you receive. It's also true that the more love you give, the more love you'll feel for yourself.

Children are living proof of this truth about love. Parenthood is a naturally transformative experience and often causes people to realize new dimensions of love and strength within themselves. As one young woman said about being a mother, "It's not the love you *get*, it's the love you *give*, that changes you."

It's natural and easy for most people to extend love to their families and romantic partners. Showing love to your loved ones is, of course, one of the most joyous and human of all experiences. But extending love, in the form of a simple, caring gesture, perhaps, to someone outside your intimate circle is also part of living a whole life. Developing compassion and empathy for someone who is difficult for you to love can build self-esteem and strengthen the mental/spiritual side of your Triangle. This shift in thinking and feeling is profoundly strengthening.

Altruism can strengthen every side of your Triangle. Dr. George E. Vaillant conducted a forty-year study of Harvard graduates, which was reported in his book *Adaptation to Life*. He found that altruism was one of the qualities that helped the men in the study group cope well with stress. A survey of one thousand people conducted by the California Department of Mental Health in 1980 and 1981 found that those who cared most for themselves and others were mentally and physically healthier than those with low concern for themselves and their fellow human beings.

OVERCOMING FEAR AND GUILT

The two worst enemies on your mental side are fear and guilt, which sap your energy and sabotage all three sides of your Holistic Triangle.

Just as you need to realize the true meaning of disease, it's also critical to understand the reality of fear. There's a saying: FEAR = False Experience Appearing Real.

Fear is fantasy and negative projection about the future. Guilt is negative fantasy about the past and its consequences in the future. If you keep bringing yourself back into the present, you can free yourself of a tremendous burden.

Your mind belongs to you. Remember, you can truly *change* your mind. You don't have to be a slave to negative thoughts and fantasies. You can project the future with hope. And you can spend more time in the present. But it takes practice and discipline. Don't be frustrated if you can't "change your mind" at first; be gentle and loving with yourself and keep trying.

The next time you start getting fearful and anxious, stop and ask yourself: What is this fear actually about? Unless you're in an extremely rare position of immediate physical danger, the fear will be about the future. The fear will be a result of projecting a negative fantasy about a future event.

Instead of getting carried away with the fantasy, bring yourself back to the present. Look around and really see where you are; feel the position of your body; listen to what you're hearing. Feel the breath coming in and out of your body. Realize that you have absolutely nothing to fear in the present. Affirm that you can exercise your free will to project the future with hope instead of fear.

Remember, you don't need fear and guilt to be safe. The less fear in your life, the more energy you'll have available for healing, positive action, and love. Fear and guilt are vampiric emotions. You don't have to let them drain your life force.

When you feel fearful or guilty, respond to this feeling by doing something to nourish your Triangle and something to help someone else. React by doing the best you can.

You can make the choice to free your body of medicines and toxic foods, and you can make the choice to free your mind of toxic emotions. The first step is to bring consciousness into your actions and thoughts.

SPIRITUAL NOURISHMENT

As long as you respect the laws of nature and the rights of other people, you're free to follow your own vision. You don't have to be a prisoner of anyone else's expectations or rules of success. You don't have to live by fear and guilt. Listen to your higher self instead of your ego.

All too often we forget to nourish our spiritual sides in the rush to succeed in the material world. But to be truly healthy and whole, we need contact with the Higher Force.

There are many names for this spiritual force: God, the Lord, the Light, the Universe, the Creator, the Higher Self, the Higher Power, the Source, Cosmic Consciousness, and countless other terms that strive to communicate what is ultimately beyond words. The ways in which people name, visualize, and seek contact with this power are as diverse as human beings themselves.

What you believe is a sacred and personal choice. I would never presume to tell you what to think or how to worship. I only want to encourage you to take the time to foster your spirituality, in whatever form it takes.

Listen to what your own heart and spirit tell you is true. "To thine own self be true." Develop and trust your own interpretation and practice of God and love. As the Bible says, "The kingdom of God is within you." Take the time and care to get in touch with the riches of your spiritual kingdom.

The two worst enemies on the spiritual side are rejection and lack of faith. Don't close yourself off to the Higher Force because of negative associations you may have with organized religion. Your spirituality is a precious gift. Choose the form and practice that make you comfortable and come from your heart.

Love, faith, and health are inextricably linked. When you feel close to your Creator, you feel love. When you have faith in a Higher Force, you believe in your inner healing power. This is a truth that can never be fully expressed in words; it can only be felt. So let's set aside the words for a moment and try an exercise to nurture your love and faith.

HEALING MOMENTS

The best place to begin your spiritual exploration is in the bathtub. This may surprise you, but if you try the following practice, you'll experience why this works.

Fill the tub only about one quarter of the way so the warm water barely covers your abdomen. Slide down so your head and back are flat on the bottom of the tub, and put your feet up against the wall or edge of the tub. This is a way to re-create the feeling of being in the womb.

If this sounds too strange at the moment, or you don't have a bathtub, you can practice Healing Moments lying on a carpet or a pad on the floor. Turn off the phone, lower the lights, and try to block out any other distractions.

Begin by inhaling slowly through your nose. Fill up your abdomen with your breath, then your rib cage and then your chest. Now exhale slowly and completely. This is diaphragmatic breathing, and it is used in most meditation practices. Establish this pattern until it becomes comfortable.

As you inhale, feel your body becoming light, floating. Slowly lift up your hands. Feel the pure white light and love of the Universe entering through your fingertips. This is the light and love of the Creator and humanity. Feel it fill you up, and absorb the love into your body, your solar plexus, your heart.

If there is a place in your body with a pain or problem, send the light-love to that spot. See and feel the healing light-love soothe and balance that area.

As you exhale, send the love and energy back out, to the Creator and to all the people in the world. Direct some of your healing light-love to specific people who need it. Send it to people you need to forgive. Keep inhaling the love, filling yourself up with it, and exhaling, sending it back out to the Universe.

When you're ready to emerge from the Healing Moment, do so gently, slowly. First open your eyes and stretch a little. Then turn to one side, and rise to a sitting position slowly.

Try to follow the Healing Moment with another nourishing activity. If you're in the tub, you can continue with the Bathing Ritual on page 219. If you're on the floor, this is a good time to do yoga or to stretch. You can turn on the light and read a book on a spiritual topic. Your mind and body are open and relaxed; be careful what stimulus you give yourself.

Now that you've read through this section, please try it.

How did it go? If you are new to any form of meditation, you may have experienced some common blocks. Maybe you felt silly or uneasy. Perhaps you felt skeptical or insincere. Perhaps your thoughts kept darting all over, and you couldn't concentrate on the healing. These all are extremely common reactions. Don't berate yourself. Just keep at the practice.

The moment will come when you truly feel the light and love. As you become more and more adept with this practice, you'll be able to evoke the feeling in different circumstances. You'll be putting together the mental and spiritual in a very powerful way.

MEDITATION IS FOR EVERYONE

Meditation is not just for yogis sitting in lotus positions in India or those with exotic lifestyles. Meditation can benefit everyone everywhere. For many years holistic healers have recognized the ability of regular meditation to reduce mind/body stress, improve mental attitude, and enhance the immune response.

In the past decade medical science has finally started to give attention to the link between mind and immunity, and this has given rise to a new discipline called psychoneuroimmunology, or PNI. Dr. Bernie Siegel, author of *Love, Medicine and Miracles*, and Dr. Joan Borysenko, author of *Minding the Body, Mending the Mind*, are two leading lights in this field.

There are many different forms and philosophies of meditation. Basically meditation is a way to quiet the mind and give yourself a respite from the usual busy thoughts. Meditation is a way to focus your mind firmly in the present moment, without thought of the future or past. It's good practice for bringing yourself back into the present to eliminate fear.

There are various types of meditation that use mantras, prayers, or religious chants as focal points. Other people prefer to use a simple word such as "one" or to concentrate on their breathing. Whichever form you practice, meditation will help you get in touch with your spiritual self. See page 183 for instructions on how to meditate.

AFFIRMATIONS

Another way to nourish your mental/spiritual side is to use affirmations, which are a form of positive programming. Affirmations involve replacing negative thought patterns with positive statements that you repeat to yourself until they become part of your reality.

You can say your affirmations out loud, repeat them to yourself silently, or write them down. Some people like to have written affirmations greet them when they open their closets or drawers. Sitting quietly and repeating the affirmations has a powerful effect, but you can also sing them to yourself while you do housework or take a walk.

Affirmations can be any positive statement, stated in the present tense. Some basic examples, which may be familiar, are:

I enjoy vibrant good health.
I love and accept every part of myself.
I have loving, nourishing relationships.
I am filled with unconditional love.

Affirmations can also be more specific, about your career, relationships, or any other aspect of your life. However, affirmations are not to be used to manipulate other people or as a selfish "wish list." The idea is to state affirmations that establish basic patterns of positive thinking and leave you open to a variety of possibilities. You don't want to turn your affirmation practice into a goal-oriented task. Leave yourself open, and use affirmations for spiritual growth.

When you compose your affirmations, make them short, clear, and positive, and state them in the present tense. For example, instead of saying, "I am not nervous or tense," say, "I am calm and relaxed." Make your affirmations about yourself, not about others. "I attract loving relationships," is preferable to "Everyone falls madly in love with me."

As you repeat your affirmations, try to let go of your doubts and judgments. Try to believe in your affirmations even if they are not reflective of your present reality.

VISUALIZATION

Visualization or positive imagery is another way to nourish the mental/spiritual side of your Triangle. Visualization, like meditation, should be done in a quiet place and a comfortable position. You begin by relaxing your body and focusing on your breath. Then you imagine a scene that nourishes your mind/body.

Another way to use visualization is for specific goals. Once you have set the goal, you begin the visualization in the same way: Sit comfortably; close your eyes; concentrate on your breath. Now imagine or see the scene in your mind.

For example, if you want to give up caffeine, picture yourself starting the day with a glass of fruit juice instead of coffee, drinking lots of refreshing mineral water, and feeling energetic yet calm all morning. If you want to handle a difficult person with more patience, you can visualize yourself responding to the person's complaints in a more compassionate manner.

The goal is to imagine the scene in great detail, to create a vivid positive image in your mind in place of a negative projection. Of course, this doesn't mean everything will always go exactly as you visualize or affirm. But it can help tremendously to use the power of your mind and the natural habit of association to create positive expectations instead of fear.

Visualization can be a powerful healing tool. It may take time and patience before you can fully utilize imagery to evoke your natural healing force, but it is an exercise that is well worth practicing. Please see page 184 for guided healing visualizations.

EXPERIMENT

This chapter has introduced you to many ways in which you can nourish your mental/spiritual side. Try a variety of techniques, and see which ones work best for you. It doesn't mean you're a spiritual dilettante if you experiment with different ways to strengthen your mental/spiritual base. However, consistency is needed for true spiritual growth. After you find the practices that feel right, try to do them on a regular basis.

Everyone has different ways to express unconditional love and nurture her or his spirituality. Your individual temperament, your lifestyle, and your religious background and upbringing all will influence your choices.

The only absolute rule is that you need to nourish this mental/ spiritual side of your Triangle to be holistically healthy. Mental/spiritual nourishment and love are as essential to good health as the food you eat. Take time to eliminate toxic fear and guilt from your mental diet and to feed yourself more love and faith.

CHAPTER 3

The Chemical Side of Your Holistic Triangle

When your body is free of toxins, an incredible healing force is released. You can think more clearly, you can take deeper breaths, and your body can gather all its energy to heal ailments that may have been plaguing you for years. It's an energizing, joyful state that you need to experience firsthand to appreciate fully.

The goal on the chemical side of the Holistic Triangle is to eliminate toxins and to increase your intake of natural, wholesome, unprocessed foods. Then you can experience for yourself the power and pleasure of detoxification.

Although nourishing all three sides of your Holistic Triangle is crucial to good health, the choices you make on the chemical side can be a matter of life and death. According to the *Surgeon General's Report on Nutrition and Health,* food can affect the risk of diseases that account for more than two thirds of all deaths in the United States: coronary heart disease, stroke, atherosclerosis, diabetes, and some types of cancer. One of the most important and life-affirming steps you can take is to improve your diet.

THE HOLISTIC FOOD GROUPS

In the spring of 1991 the U.S. Department of Agriculture was set to issue a pamphlet titled *U.S.D.A.'s Eating Right Pyramid*. The meat and dairy interests were upset that their products were given less space on the pyramid than grains, fruits, and vegetables were. In fact, meat and dairy products merited just slightly more space than fats and sweets. Pressure from meat and dairy industry groups held up the release of the food pyramid for another year.

The new food pyramid, which was finally released by the USDA is a step in the right direction since it suggests fewer servings of meat and eggs and more of vegetable and grain products. But it is a timid step that does not go nearly far enough in giving Americans optimal nutritional advice. The pyramid recommends two to three servings of milk, yogurt, or cheese, whereas eliminating dairy products altogether is a better idea for most people. And the pyramid fails to emphasize that the bread, cereal, rice, or pasta products should be whole grains and unrefined forms of these foods. The Holistic Food Pyramid on page 49 represents a better balance for optimal nourishment and detoxification.

HEALTHY ALTERNATIVES TO THE TOP TEN TOXINS

Strengthening the chemical side of your Holistic Triangle boils down to a simple formula: *Less toxic input; more wholesome input.*

The Top Ten Toxins are substances that weaken your Holistic Triangle: sugar, white flour and other refined carbohydrates, dairy products, meat, food additives, nicotine, caffeine, alcohol, drugs, and environmental toxins.

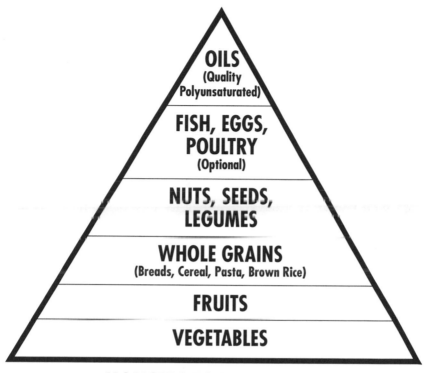

HOLISTIC FOOD PYRAMID

The goal is to eliminate these toxins from your *daily* diet. If you choose to have a cappuccino on a sunny day in Little Italy, eat roast beef on Christmas, or drink a glass of champagne during a romantic dinner, it's not going to do you a great deal of harm. It's the habits you indulge in day after day, year after year—the ones that your own body tells you it wants to dispense with—that you need to address.

Certain toxins, such as nicotine, you'll need to eliminate completely and forever. Other substances on this list, such as alcohol, sugar, and meat, you may want to indulge in occasionally. The choice is yours, but it's important you have enough knowledge to make intelligent decisions.

Entire books have been written to explain the hazards of many of these toxins. If you have an addiction to a particular substance, such as sugar, and have a hard time believing you need to give it up, you might do additional reading on your pet poison. Meanwhile, the information here will alert you to some of the dangers. The purpose of this section is not to scare you; it's to motivate you to make changes. I've provided healthy alternatives to each toxin to show you'll be gaining more than you give up.

Sugar

Understand that sugar is a drug. Large amounts of refined sugar have a profound physiological response and pharmacological effect. A "sweet tooth" is a euphemism for "sugar addiction."

It's well known that sugar is a major cause of tooth decay and causes overweight. Sugar provides virtually no vitamins, minerals, enzymes, or any other nutrients. Sugar actually *drains* the body of vitamins and minerals, while placing a tremendous strain on its systems.

Most of us are familiar with the sugar "buzz" and subsequent letdown. Sugar can produce an emotional roller coaster: anxiety, shakiness, and other metabolic responses culminating in the "sugar blues." These reactions reflect what refined sugar does to your blood sugar level.

Sugar consumption causes the blood sugar to rise rapidly. The pancreas responds by churning out insulin, which causes the blood sugar level to fall. These sharp fluctuations can lead to anxiety and depression. As with other addictions, the sugar "high" is followed by a crash.

Worse yet is the long-term effect: stress on the adrenals and endocrine system that can lead to hypoglycemia and diabetes. Studies by Dr. Thomas Cleve (the former surgeon captain of the Royal Navy and research director of the British Institute of Naval Medicine) found that increases in consumption of sugar and refined carbohydrates in residents of African nations were followed by precipitous rises in diabetes cases in these countries.

A warning is needed about products that are falsely presented as safe substitutes for sugar. Brown sugar is simply white sugar with a small amount of molasses added for coloring. Molasses is a by-product of sugar refining and is also nutritionally worthless.

The "sugar substitutes" cooked up in laboratories are far worse. In fact, you're probably better off consuming plain old white sugar than artificial sweeteners.

After a two-year investigation of aspartame, the Government Accounting Office (GAO) reported that 40 percent of the scientists surveyed called for further research, 32 percent suggested new warnings, and 15 percent favored a total ban of the sweetener. Studies reported in the *Tufts University School of Nutrition Guide to Total Nutrition* found that large amounts of saccharin cause bladder cancer in laboratory animals.

The data on artificial sweeteners are incomplete, and more carcinogenic effects may be found in the future. Remember that cyclamates were an approved sweetener for twenty-five years until they were found to cause bladder tumors in lab rats and finally banned in 1969.

Healthy Alternatives

There are some natural sweeteners that are safe if used sparingly. Raw, unheated, unfiltered honey and maple syrup in small amounts are acceptable. Barley malt syrup is a grain-based sweetener that has less impact on the body than refined sugar. Rice syrup is another gentle sweetener.

The healthiest sweetness comes from the sun, in all the wonderfully diverse forms of fruits. Fruit juices are versatile sweeteners to use in cooking and baking. Fruit itself is the healthiest sweet snack. Fruit juices are nutritious sweet beverages, but they should always be diluted with 50 percent water to reduce the fructose concentration. Fructose in other forms should be used sparingly.

White Flour and Refined Carbohydrates

Nature produces a miniature nutritional miracle in each tiny grain. Unfortunately, modern food processing strips away most of the nutrients and leaves empty calories.

Whole wheat contains essential amino acids, fiber, vitamins, minerals, and trace elements. But nearly all these nutrients are found in the germ and bran layers, which are removed to produce white flour. Processing also strips rice of its most nutritious layers to produce white rice.

White flour and polished rice, and foods made from their ingredients, are lacking in B vitamins and can exacerbate B deficiency. In addition, altering the form of complex carbohydrates through food processing affects the rate of digestion and absorption and can lead to blood sugar level problems.

Healthy Alternatives

Instead of nutritionally deficient white flour products, you can choose from a great variety of whole grain foods.

—Whole wheat flour is the most popular choice for cooking. You can also use buckwheat flour, rice flour, rye flour, and cornmeal for different recipes. Many prepared baked goods are now made with these whole grain flours. (A small amount of white flour may be included in these products.)
—Brown rice still has the germ and bran layers intact and is far more nutritious and satisfying than white rice. Wild rice, which is actually the seed of an aquatic grass, has a distinctive taste and texture.
—Dried pastas made from whole wheat flour are available, some with vegetables such as spinach, carrots, and tomatoes added. Japanese soba noodles, made from buckwheat and wheat flour, are a tasty option.
—A wide selection of hot and cold cereals is made from whole grains. Look for products sweetened with fruit juice instead of sugar.

You can also expand your grain repertoire far beyond rice. Bulgur, traditionally used in Middle Eastern cooking, is a precooked grain with a nutty flavor. Couscous made from whole wheat flour is another idea. Millet can be eaten as a breakfast cereal or used in other meals instead of rice. Amaranth and quinoa have been called supergrains because of their high nutrient content. A selection of fascinating health food cookbooks can teach you how to prepare these and other grains.

Dairy Products

The National Dairy Council does a tremendous job convincing Americans of two lies: Milk is essential for children, and dairy products are also healthy for adults. The milk myth is one of the most widespread examples of nutritional brainwashing. Even baby calves can't survive on homogenized milk, yet we feed our children cow's milk loaded with antibiotics, synthetic hormones, and pesticide and herbicide residues.

The consumption of milk, cheese, butter, and other dairy products has been found by researchers to be a factor in atherosclerosis, heart attacks, and strokes. One of the largest studies of diet and health ever undertaken was the China-Oxford-Cornell Project on Nutrition, Health, and the Environment (also known as the China Health Project), begun in 1983 and reported upon in 1990. This study found both dairy and meat consumption is unnecessary and can contribute to cancer, heart disease, obesity, and many other illnesses.

In addition to the problems caused by high-fat content, dairy products contain alarmingly high levels of pesticide residues and other environmental contaminants. Compounding this danger is the high level of antibiotics in cattle feed, which becomes concentrated in dairy products and meat.

Dairy products are also a leading cause of food allergies. At about the age of four many people begin to lose the ability to digest lactose, which is the carbohydrate found in milk. Lactose intolerance is particularly high in certain ethnic groups, including Asians, African Americans, and Jews. Allergies to milk caseinate, or protein, are also common. Symptoms of dairy allergy can include irritability, muscle pain, mental depression, abdominal pain, cramps, gas, diarrhea, constipation, nasal stuffiness, and sinusitis. For more on detecting dairy and other food allergies, see page 194.

Yogurt is promoted as a health food, but this is another illusion created by clever marketers. Most supermarket brands of yogurt contain sugar and milk from polluted American cattle and are a far different substance from the natural product that helps people live to be one hundred and five in the Caucasus Mountains.

If you want to eat yogurt, do so in moderation, and be sure to choose a type with active yogurt cultures and without added sugar. Or, if possible, make your own yogurt with milk from an organic farm.

Healthy Alternatives

The delicious, nutritious alternatives to cow's milk include soy beverage, almond beverage, and rice beverage. These can be used in cereal, for cooking, or as satisfying drinks.

Margarine is *not* a healthy substitute for butter since it is hydrogenated and can interfere with the body's ability to absorb calcium and magnesium. Alternatives include almond butter, filbert butter, cashew butter, pecan butter, and apple butter.

Health food stores now offer cholesterol-free "mayonnaise" made from tofu. Soy cheeses and yogurts are also available.

Despite what the Dairy Council would have us believe, human beings *do not* need cow's milk or cheese for calcium. Calcium comes from soil and is absorbed into the structure of plants. That's how cattle get calcium. Why not get the calcium directly from the source instead of filtered through a contaminated cow?

Foods with high levels of calcium include green vegetables, such as kale and spinach; fish, beans, and nuts; and soy beverages fortified with vitamins, minerals, and protein.

Meat

For decades, nutritionists and cardiologists have urged Americans to eat less meat to avoid heart attacks, strokes, and cancer. Thousands of articles have been published demonstrating that the less animal fat you take into your body, the healthier you will be. Even the usually conservative American Dietetic Association came out with a paper that stated people who do not consume meat are at a lower risk for colon cancer, heart disease, obesity, adult-onset diabetes, high blood pressure, osteoporosis, kidney stones, gallstones, breast cancer, and lung cancer.

In 1990 the *New England Journal of Medicine* reported the results of a survey of the health and diet histories of more than eighty-eight thousand women. This survey found that the more red meat and animal fat the women ate, the more likely they were to develop cancer of the colon. Cancers of the prostate, kidneys, testicles, uterus, lungs, and breasts and lymphomas are also higher in populations that consume diets high in fat.

Animal flesh contains high levels of environmental contaminants, which are ingested by animals and concentrated in their fatty tissues. Meat is further contaminated by hormones, stimulants, and antibiotics used to speed animal growth and combat infectious illness. Many of these contaminants have been found or are suspected of causing cancers, birth defects, and other severe effects.

Switching to a vegetarian diet can help save the planet as well as yourself. Beef production accounts for an enormous waste of land that could be more efficiently utilized for grain production. According to John Robbins, author of *Diet for a New America* and *May All Be Fed*, if Americans reduced their meat consumption by only 10 percent, it would free land and resources to grow more than twelve million tons of grain each year and feed forty to sixty million people. As the population of the planet continues to explode, we desperately need to shift to an agriculture that feeds people, not livestock.

If you are sincerely concerned about the destruction of the tropical rain forest, you'll want to give up beef since much of the rain forest is razed to give way to cattle-grazing land. Throughout the world more and more forests are being cut down to clear land for grazing or growing cattle feed. By reducing the demand for meat, we can help curb the destruction of the environment.

Healthy Alternatives

Nature provides a bounty of foods that contain high levels of protein without the side effects of meat and dairy products. The vegetable foods with the highest protein levels are legumes—that is, beans, peas, and lentils.

It is *not* necessary to combine foods to "create" complete proteins, as some early vegetarian books suggested. Legumes and other high-protein plant foods are sufficient sources of protein by themselves. However, several different types of plant protein should be consumed in the course of a week.

Tofu, made from soybeans, is a favorite with vegetarian cooks because it has a neutral taste that soaks up seasonings and sauces. It comes in firm and soft forms and can be baked, broiled, grilled, marinated, scrambled, or steamed for use in salads, dressings, soups, main dishes, and desserts. Tempeh, which is also made from soybeans, has a rich, meatlike taste when it is prepared with the right seasonings.

Nuts and seeds are also high in protein, but they need to be eaten in moderation because they are high in calories. Buy and eat nuts in their natural form—that is, unsalted and raw—rather than roasted. Roasted nuts have already been cooked, and the oils within the nuts hydrogenated, so your body cannot utilize the oils as effectively.

Other high- to medium-high-protein foods include potatoes, corn, oatmeal, onions, artichokes, asparagus, mushrooms, spinach, kale, lettuce (except iceberg), and oranges.

A Word About Fish, Chicken, and Eggs

A vegetarian diet with careful attention to eating enough protein foods is the purest and most nourishing plan for the chemical side of your Holistic Triangle. It also provides the steady energy you need for a vigorous physical side.

From the mental/spiritual standpoint, practitioners of spiritual disciplines usually advocate a vegetarian diet for two reasons. First of all, it's obviously more humane not to have any living creatures killed for your supper. Secondly, meat is dense food that requires a lot of energy in the gastrointestinal tract to break down. It tends to create a lethargic mental state that makes concentration more difficult.

However, sticking to a vegetarian diet may be too much of an adjustment for you at this time. If this is the case, it's recommended you give up red meat and consume fish, eggs, and chicken in moderation.

Fish would be a healthy food if we lived in a pristine world. Unfortunately our rivers, lakes, and oceans are highly polluted, and their poisons accumulate in the fish tissues. Shellfish carry particularly high levels of toxic lead, cadmium, arsenic, and other heavy metals, along with dangerous microbes and toxins. Shellfish are also a cause of frequent food allergies and should be avoided entirely. Stick with fish high in omega fatty acids, such as haddock, halibut, salmon, and swordfish. Always select the fish carefully, and eat it cooked, not raw.

If you choose to eat chicken, purchase only free-range chicken from health food stores or specialty markets. Commercial chickens are raised in appalling conditions and are often contaminated. Always cook your chicken thoroughly, and again, limit the amount you eat.

If you want to eat eggs, buy brown fertilized organic eggs from your health food store. Poach or soft-boil the eggs, and try to limit yourself to two to four per week.

Food Additives

According to *Fit for Life* nutrition experts Harvey and Marilyn Diamond, more than one billion pounds of chemicals are added to food consumed by Americans each year. These include colorings, preservatives, flavoring agents, and chemicals for texture, firmness, thickening, and emulsifying. Manufacturers also add artificially produced nutrients in an attempt to replace what was destroyed by food processing.

These food additives are a frequent source of food allergies and allergic reactions. Reactions can include hyperactivity in children, weakness and fatigue, swelling, asthma, shock, headaches, and nausea.

Table salt is perhaps the most common food additive. Many people paralyze their taste buds by adding salt to everything. Eliminating this excess salt is instrumental in controlling high blood pressure and water retention.

There is enough natural salt in wholesome foods that using the shaker shouldn't be necessary. But when healthy recipes do call for salt, use a dash of sea salt.

Healthy Alternatives

The alternative to food additives is simple: Eat fresh food in its natural state, and learn to use herbs and spices in creative ways in cooking. When you do want to eat a premade bread, cereal, or snack food, check the label. If salt is one of the first ingredients listed or there are chemical additives, leave it in the store. As you lose your taste for packaged and refined foods, you'll gain a greater appreciation of the taste of the flavor of raw food in its fresh original state.

Caffeine

Nearly half the adult population of the United States is addicted to this insidious drug, which is found in coffee, tea, and many carbonated beverages. Sodas contain the double whammy of caffeine with sugar or artificial sweeteners.

Although caffeine is accepted in society, it can have serious consequences. High levels of caffeine consumption can cause nervous symptoms, including insomnia, irritability, and trembling; irritation to the stomach and diarrhea; and aggravation of heart and artery disorders.

In addition, studies have found that eliminating caffeine can control or cure fibrocystic breast disease (painful breast lumps). Even in small or moderate doses, caffeine can prevent iron from being properly utilized and cause other vitamins to be pumped through the body before they are absorbed.

Caffeine is a stimulant, and what goes up must come down. The surge of mental energy is often followed by a letdown, leading to an urge for another dose. This creates the cycle of caffeine addiction.

Decaffeinated beverages are *not* recommended since the process of decaffeination is itself questionable. Methylene chloride, which is used to extract the caffeine from coffee beans by some companies, has been found to cause cancer when inhaled in large amounts by laboratory animals. Even when other decaf methods are used, you'll be making a more health-affirming choice by leaving the beverage behind altogether.

Healthy Alternatives

Maintaining a good energy level through good nutrition, adequate rest, and exercise is the best substitute for caffeine. Since caffeine is highly addictive, kicking it can be hard, with low-grade headaches and fatigue common during the first days of withdrawal. But after the withdrawal is complete, your energy level should be better than ever if you nourish your Holistic Triangle well.

Increasing your oxygen consumption through exercise is the ultimate natural stimulant. Yet we need balance to be healthy, and rest is equally important. Listen to your body's signals; don't keep forcing and stressing yourself beyond natural limits.

Healthy beverage substitutes for coffee include drinks made from roasted grains and seeds. Herbal teas generally don't contain caffeine and are available in an array of flavors. You can make your own caffeine- and sugar-free soft drinks with a mixture of seltzer and fruit juice. Fruit juice, especially the type you make yourself in your juicer, can provide a natural lift.

Nicotine

It is common knowledge that nicotine addiction is a lethal habit and a leading cause of heart disease and some types of cancer. If you smoke, you probably don't need to be convinced it's bad for you.

What you need to do is take a holistic approach to kicking the habit. This requires a quit-smoking program that addresses the mental/spiritual component of the habit as well as the chemical addiction.

Healthy Alternatives

There is no healthy alternative to nicotine except to quit smoking. Breathing pure oxygen is the only substitute. Oxygen is the most important nutrient on the chemical side; it is life itself. Don't inhale death instead of life.

There are many different ways to kick the nicotine habit. Some people swear by quitting cold turkey on their own, while others find support groups and smoking-cessation clinics to be the answer. Whatever approach you take, good nutrition, plenty of exercise, and practicing relaxation methods will help you maintain your resolve.

Raw-juice fasting can be an excellent tool when you want to quit smoking. Once the body has been cleansed of accumulated poisons, the craving for nicotine often disappears. Acupuncture is an excellent aid during the nicotine withdrawal process. Some people find hypnosis helpful.

You should also be careful of the dangers of secondhand smoke. If you live or work with smokers, assert your right to a smoke-free environment. If you can't escape the smoke, supplements of vitamins A, E, and C and beta-carotene may be somewhat protective.

Alcohol

Excessive drinking can lead to alcoholism and a host of potentially fatal health problems: brain deterioration, cirrhosis of the liver, malnutrition, and strokes, as well as automobile accidents.

Even in moderation, alcohol adds empty calories and causes weight gain while it depletes vitamins. Alcohol turns into acid aldehyde, a metabolic waste product, and travels through the entire systematic circulation, burning out brain cells and causing other damage along the way. Another complication is caused by the sugar in alcohol, which can lead to or aggravate hypoglycemia.

Healthy Alternatives

Alcoholism is a disease that needs to be fought on all levels: mental/spiritual, physical, and chemical. Alcoholics Anonymous has incredible impact with its meetings, which focus on the mental/spiritual side.

Recovering alcoholics also need to pay attention to the chemical sides of their Triangles. Studies have shown that alcoholics who consume nutritious food and multivitamin supplements have greater success in staying sober. Since many heavy drinkers are also hypoglycemic, avoiding sugar and caffeine and eating small, frequent meals are recommended. Alcohol drinkers need vitamin/mineral supplementation to replace depleted nutrients. Some experts believe that supplements of L-glutamine lessen the urge to drink.

Learning to unwind without alcohol can reduce the desire to drink. Relaxation techniques, meditation, exercise, and enjoying the outdoors can take the edge off your day without the side effects of alcohol.

Many beverages can substitute for alcoholic drinks. Fruit juices mixed with carbonated water are refreshing spritzers. Sparkling cider can substitute for champagne. Punches made with blends of exotic juices and fresh fruits are festive drinks.

Drugs

The government and the media focus on the dangers of illegal drugs, such as heroin, cocaine, amphetamines, barbiturates, and hallucinogens, and most people are well aware it's wise to avoid these substances. But we need to raise our consciousness about the legal drugs that are sanctioned by the government and promoted by pharmaceutical companies.

According to Dr. Joseph Beasley, the director of Bard College's Institute of Health Policy and Practice and a leading expert in addiction, every year Americans consume more than *five billion* legal yet addictive "minor" tranquilizers for anxiety and sleeplessness.

These tranquilizers include the most popular brand names consumed by basically healthy people without severe psychological problems. Yet the side effects of these ubiquitous drugs can include drowsiness, fatigue, lack of muscle coordination, confusion, depression, headache, sleep disturbances, urinary difficulties, loss of balance, blurred vision, anxiety, and addiction.

The overuse of penicillin is another epidemic of drug abuse. Antibiotics wipe out the friendly germs in your body, especially in your digestive tract. This can allow yeasts, such as *Candida albicans*, to proliferate and put toxins into your system, leading to such potential problems as fatigue, headaches, depression, and fungal infections. The long-range effect of the frequent use of antibiotics is still in dispute, but overall lowered immune function may be the result in many cases.

Even such a "harmless" nonprescription drug as aspirin can upset the gastrointestinal tract, cause hemorrhage, stomach cramps, nausea, heartburn, and blood in the stool. Prolonged use or large doses of aspirin can result in reduced production of blood cells, kidney damage, and activation of peptic ulcer. Aspirin is a prostaglandin inhibitor, and studies have shown that long-term use can exacerbate arthritis. Decongestants, when overused, can increase blood pressure and affect circulation.

Virtually all drugs, legal or not, can have side effects, and we need to treat them as toxins that should be used only as last resorts, not as cure-alls that can be popped without concern.

Healthy Alternatives

The more you nourish the three sides of your Holistic Triangle, the less likely you are to feel the need for drugs of any kind: recreational, prescription, or over-the-counter.

On the mental/spiritual side, meditation, positive visualization and affirmation, and spiritual/religious practices can help reduce the craving for drugs.

On the chemical side, eating natural foods and avoiding toxins will help you maintain good health and reduce the need for drug remedies. Supplements also help maintain health independence from drugs. Herbal remedies can be used to treat some ailments, on a limited, short-term basis.

On the physical side of the Triangle, exercise lowers the desire for drugs by creating a natural high. Yoga and relaxation practices can reduce anxiety and create a more balanced state of mind.

Environmental Toxins

There are several categories of environmental toxins to consider: pesticides and herbicides in food, toxins in personal products, and chemicals in the home and workplace. While environmental toxins are difficult to avoid in today's world, there are many measures you can take to protect yourself and your family.

Healthy Alternatives to Pesticides and Herbicides

Fear of pesticides and herbicides should never keep you from eating plenty of fruits and vegetables since the benefits far outweigh the risks. And there are measures you can take to protect your health.

Try to purchase organic fruits and vegetables that are certified as having been grown without pesticides and herbicides. These are available in many health food stores, in special sections at some supermarkets, and at some farmers' markets (although you need to check with the growers).

If your local food store does not carry organic fruits and vegetables, speak to the manager about stocking an organic produce section, and have your friends and neighbors add their support for this idea. Another possibility is to start a health food co-op in your area.

Organic produce tends to be more expensive than the supermarket variety that is grown with pesticides and herbicides. However, in the long run organic produce supplies better value for your dollar since it has more nutrients and you don't have to discard outer layers to get rid of the poisons. You'll also save a great deal of money by switching from a meat-based to a primarily vegetarian diet.

If you are unable to obtain organic produce, choose seasonal fruits and vegetables. Avoid imported produce from countries where pesticides are not regulated stringently. If possible, buy from farmers' markets, where the produce often has less pesticides.

You can soak the produce in filtered water with vinegar and lemon juice added, or use a biodegradable vegetable rinse, available in health food stores. Always wash the produce carefully, and if it is not organic and the skin is going to be eaten, scrub it with a vegetable brush.

If you have the time, space, and inclination, growing your own fruits, vegetables, and herbs is a wonderful way to get pure produce and exercise at the same time. Gardening nourishes all three sides of your Triangle: It provides exercise on the physical side, contact with nature to nourish your mental/spiritual side, and fresh foods to strengthen your chemical side.

Avoid the use of chemical pesticides, herbicides, and fertilizers on your lawn as well as your garden. Organic gardening manuals explain natural alternatives to chemicals.

Healthy Alternatives to Toxins in the Home and Workplace

Although it is difficult to completely avoid the toxins that infiltrate our world, there are measures you can take to minimize exposure.

—Use natural cosmetics, bath products, moisturizers, soaps, deodorants, and toothpastes. These are available in health food stores, in some drugstores, and through catalogs.

—Use toxin-free household cleaners and laundry products.

—Test your home for radon. If necessary, seal cracks in foundations and floors, improve ventilation, and treat contaminated water from private wells.

—Remove existing lead paint from your home. Test tap water for lead.

—Use stainless steel instead of aluminum cookware.

—If you must use toxic chemicals for home renovations, crafts, or hobbies, work in a very well-ventilated area and limit exposure time.

—If you work in a large office building, insist on good ventilation and windows that can be opened. If you notice a number of similar sicknesses in your office, bring it to the attention of management. Band together with your coworkers, and demand an investigation into whether there is a "sick building" problem. Assert your right to have renovations done that will ensure a clean work environment.

—If you are an industrial worker, consult with your colleagues and union leaders about steps to reduce exposure to hazardous materials and toxins.

—If your job entails unavoidable exposure to toxins, you may need to consider looking for other work. Despite economic difficulties and other serious considerations, you must put your health first. Sticking with an unhealthy job can finally result in greater financial hardship from missing work as the result of illness and from large medical bills.

WATER

Water, after oxygen, is the most essential nutrient on the chemical side. Yet few of us drink enough water each day.

Drinking eight glasses of liquid each day is optimal. Some of this liquid can be diluted fruit juice, soy or nut milk, or herbal tea, but six glasses a day should be pure water. Try to have a glass of water with you throughout the day—except when you are eating.

No animal in nature eats and drinks at the same time, and neither should humans. Drinking water neutralizes the enzymatic ability of the gastric juices, hydrochloric acid and pepsin, in your stomach. Diluting your gastric juices interferes with efficient digestion and assimilation of nutrients. Therefore, it's recommended you drink most of your water between, not during, meals.

When you're drinking a lot of water, you want it to be pure. But water straight from the tap cannot be trusted in most cities and towns. Many people drink bottled water, which usually comes in a plastic rather than a glass container. The drawbacks to bottled water are the plastic residue and the impact on the environment from all those discarded plastic bottles and jugs. A better solution is to purchase a water filter to attach directly to your tap. Then you can use pure water for your cooking as well as straight drinking. Having a water cooler with delivery of fresh springwater in reusable jugs is another option.

A HEALTHFUL DIET

The sun is our original source of energy, and foods that thrive on sunlight and soil provide energy. When you eat more live foods, you feel more alive.

Revitalizing the chemical side of your Triangle is an opportunity to enjoy more of nature's bounty and reject civilization's poisons. This is part of creating your own paradise. You won't go hungry in the "Garden of Eden," but you will have to detoxify to get there.

When you're radically changing your nourishment on the chemical side of your Triangle, it helps to have reinforcement on the mental/spiritual side by reading books on nutrition and health food cooking. By educating yourself about natural food, you'll learn that the choices of healthy nourishment are varied and enticing. See page 187 for Healthful Meal Plan guidelines.

You'll notice this plan consists of six meals, not three. It's not just what you eat; it's what you *assimilate* that strengthens your Triangle. Eating small, frequent meals provides a steady stream of nutrients without overtaxing your digestive system. This eating plan facilitates the ability of digestive enzymes to break down complex molecules into simple ones your body can absorb.

It's important to chew all your food slowly and thoroughly to maximize assimilation of nutrients. Chewing does more than break up food so you can gulp it down; it stimulates the production of digestive juices.

You can create the right frame of mind to appreciate your food by taking a few seconds to calm down before you eat. Close your eyes, take a few deep breaths, and give thanks to the Universe for your nourishment.

INDIVIDUALIZED NEEDS

When designing a healthy diet for yourself, consider your ethnic background and your genetic predisposition. Everyone is different, and while there are general guidelines, it's best to adapt your diet to suit your individuality. To accomplish this, you need to consider both your ancestry and your present way of life.

For example, if you have a heavy manual job, you can utilize more calories and larger portions than if you sit at a desk. If you are very athletic, you can also increase your intake. Your body size, build, and metabolism are factors. You may need to experiment with the amount of food you eat to lose or maintain a desirable weight as you adapt your diet.

Many people find they lose weight on a natural-food six-small-meals-a-day plan. The trick is to eat smaller portions of a variety of high-energy foods. This helps prevent your craving high-calorie foods and keeps your metabolism going at a brisk pace. It's especially helpful to eat lightly after sundown.

You can also use food as a targeted therapeutic tool to heal specific diseases and ailments. Nutritionists specialize in designing customized diets to treat health problems. There are many fine books on using foods for healing, in which you can look up your ailment and get a food prescription. This is another example of how strengthening the mental side of the Triangle can heal the chemical and physical sides.

A DOZEN HEALTHY EATING HINTS

- Just because a product is sold in a health food store doesn't mean it's healthy. Watch out for products containing too much honey, fructose, corn syrup, and oil.
- Fill your shopping basket with organic fruits and vegetables.
- Buy grains, nuts, and seeds from bag-it-yourself bins in health food stores to save money.
- Find out if there is a health food store co-op, owned and operated by customers, in your area. Food co-ops can be very economical, and you might consider organizing one if you have the time and interest.
- Use only small amounts of high-quality, cold-pressed, poly-

unsaturated oils for cooking and salad dressings: flaxseed oil, olive oil, safflower oil, and sunflower oil.

- Eat fruits and vegetables in their raw state whenever possible. When you do cook vegetables, steam them instead of boiling or sautéing them.
- Prepare green salads shortly before mealtimes, and use leafy green types of lettuce but no iceberg lettuce. If you're eating salad with other foods, have it during or after the meal, not before.
- Increase fiber by choosing only whole grains cereals, pastas, and breads. Add bran to cereals and batters.
- Prepare your lunch and snacks to take to work, so you know you'll be eating nutritious, pure food.
- Make your food preferences known ahead of time when you are eating at a friend's or relative's house. If you think this is imposing, offer to bring your own meal.
- Share your reasons for eliminating toxins and eating natural foods with your family, but don't shove your choices down their throats or expect them to see the light overnight.
- In addition to natural food restaurants, ethnic restaurants often have many vegetable-based entrées. Assert yourself in restaurants, and ask them to prepare what you want, how you want it.

WHAT GOES IN MUST COME OUT

Frequent bowel movements are a vital element of your holistic health regimen since partially digested food builds up in the bowel and can cause toxicity and disease. You'll find that giving up toxins and eating more fruits, vegetables, and grains will result in easier elimination, although it may take time for your body to adjust.

You can add flaxseed or bran to juice or cereals for more help. A recipe for a special Fiber Broth to aid elimination is on page 193. Drinking eight glasses of water a day also alleviates constipation. Supplements of probiotic microorganisms (e.g. acidophilus) can provide healthy intestinal flora, which may be lacking.

Since eating stimulates the peristaltic action of a healthy bowel, the best time for a bowel movement is after a meal. Avoid reading and other distractions when you're on the toilet; relax and allow your mind/body to focus on its natural response.

The modern toilet bowl does us a great disservice. The bowls are too high up and removed from the natural squatting position. Squatting increases intra-abdominal pressure and creates more compression and force in the bowel to get rid of the stool. It also improves the tone of intestinal muscles. You can modify the toilet bowl by placing a small stool (pardon the pun) under your feet to elevate your knees.

RAW-JUICE FASTING

One of the most powerful tools on the chemical side of the Holistic Triangle is raw-juice fasting. Fasting has been used since antiquity as a healing method. It has a profound effect on the mental/spiritual side as well as the chemical side and is part of many spiritual traditions. People often associate fasting with deprivation and starvation. Raw-juice fasting, however, is quite the opposite and can supply more nutrients than the Standard American Diet.

Raw-juice fasting can have dramatic effects on chronic problems. Brenda, a woman in her mid-thirties, had frequent constipation and chronic cystitis. Three or four times a year the cystitis would flare up and her doctor would put her on antibiotics. By the time she came to the Holistic Health Force, she needed very strong antibiotics to get temporary relief. Taking these antibiotics on a regular basis weakened her immune system and made her vulnerable to yeast infections.

Brenda's Holistic Self-Health Program began with cutting out toxins, particularly red meat, which she ate frequently. Eliminating meat and refined foods and consuming more raw foods, juices, and water solved her problem with constipation.

Two months after eliminating toxins from her diet (except for occasional lapses), Brenda was ready to embark on a three-day raw-juice fast. The fast cleaned out the lingering toxins in her system, and she immediately felt lighter and more energetic. After the discipline of the juice fast, she had more resolution to begin eliminating other toxins. She also decided to go on a raw-juice fast once each season. Brenda hasn't had a single episode of cystitis in more than three years.

Even people who are in good health and have nutritious diets can benefit from raw-juice fasting. Danny, a graphic designer in his late twenties, was a healthy eater but liked to party and stay out late drinking with his friends. He had started to gain weight around the middle and sometimes lacked energy and had difficulty concentrating.

Danny found that during and after his raw-juice fast he was mentally stimulated and unusually creative. He also lost weight and was energized to get serious about exercise. Now Danny goes on a juice fast two or three times a year because he enjoys the enhanced clarity, vigor, and creativity.

For more information on raw-juice fasting and instructions on how to use this healing force, see page 188.

SUPPLEMENTS AND HERBS

If the planet were still fresh and unpolluted, it would be possible to get all the vitamins, minerals, and enzymes we need from food. Sadly much of the soil in which today's produce is grown is depleted, and modern farming methods cause further depletion. While it is vital to consume plenty of fresh fruits and vegetables, we also need to supplement our diets to have optimal nourishment. See page 196 for information on choosing supplements.

As well as provide a backbone of basic strength and strong immunity, supplements can be used for specific therapeutic purposes. The chart on page 197 provides details about the specific properties of different vitamins and minerals.

Herbs have been used since ancient times for healing, prevention, and health maintenance. Eastern systems of medicine and folk healers throughout the world have used herbs throughout the centuries, and now holistic doctors continue the tradition. See page 205 for a summary of herbs with special healing properties.

CHAPTER 4

The Physical Side
of Your Holistic Triangle

Health is a consummation of a love affair with the organs of the
body.

—PLATO

Your physical state is an outward reflection of the amount of love
and nourishment you give the three sides of your Holistic Triangle. Genetics play an important role, but your actions are also instrumental on the physical side. And since you can't change your
genetic legacy, there's no use "blaming" it for physical limitations.
The healthiest response is to accept and love what you were
given as you work to strengthen your physical side.

There are three basic forms of nourishment on the physical
side:

- Primary physical nourishment, which you give to yourself.
  This is the most important form of nourishment and includes exercise, relaxation, and rest.
- Secondary physical nourishment, which is provided by holistic practitioners. This includes chiropractic care, massage,
  exercise instruction, and many other natural therapies.
- Tertiary physical care, which is given by medical doctors
  and includes surgical procedures.

Surgery can be lifesaving in cases of injury and severe degenerative conditions, and medical doctors should be applauded for the valuable work they perform. However, the holistic viewpoint is that surgery should be utilized selectively and carefully, in emergency situations and when limitations of matter inhibit natural healing.

We should not count on surgeons to "fix" our bodies as if they are repairmen and we are machines. We need to do everything we can to nurture and love our bodies into health before resorting to invasive procedures. The more we nourish the physical side of our Triangles, the less likely we are to end up on the operating table.

AEROBIC EXERCISE

There are three main categories of exercise: aerobic exercise, which works the cardiovascular system; musculoskeletal development, which builds the muscles; and stretching, which provides flexibility. A basic holistic exercise program consists of alternating at least three days of aerobics and three days of musculoskeletal development and of stretching every day. Adding days of aerobic exercise is fine, and you may find that some activities combine the aerobic and musculoskeletal workouts.

Aerobic exercise tones the muscles and conditions the heart to pump more blood with each stroke. This results in a lowered resting heart rate and better cardiovascular fitness, which can lower the risk of heart disease. A fifteen-year study at the Institute for Aerobics Research in Texas found definite links between physical activity and life expectancy.

One of the goals of aerobic exercise is to oxygenate your body by forcing a large volume of blood through your heart, lungs, and muscle groups. Your breath should flow with each repetition of the aerobic movement. Inhale through your nose, and exhale through your mouth or nose, and keep breathing steadily throughout the workout.

Exercising with a holistic attitude allows aerobics to nourish the mental/spiritual as well as the physical side of your Triangle. Although it's fine to set exercise goals, try not to be entirely goal-oriented. Enjoy the process, not just racing to the finish line. Wellness, not winning or making another mile, is the ultimate goal. Don't judge your performance; congratulate yourself for trying. Anything you do to nourish your physical side means you're winning!

With the right attitude, aerobic exercise can relieve tension and strengthen your stress-coping mechanisms. When you have a well-conditioned cardiovascular system, your heart rate still rises under stress, but not as high or as quickly as that of a person who is not fit. This "ceiling" on the heart rate can enable you to stay calmer during periods of stress and reduce the chance of sudden heart attack.

Regular exercise is likely to improve your self-image and boost your confidence. Many people report that during and after brisk exercise they feel more able to cope with the demands of their lives; they feel strong and "on top of the world." Studies have shown that people who exercise have more positive images of their bodies than people who don't. Of course, this improved self-image is grounded in reality since exercise helps you look better to the rest of your world as well as to yourself.

During aerobic exercise, increased blood flow to the brain can boost your thinking power. Studies have shown aerobic exercise can improve memory, verbal fluency, and creative problem solving. This effect is enhanced by the rhythmic nature of aerobics, which induces a tranquil yet lucid state of mind.

"Runner's high" is a misnomer since this sensation of euphoria is also enjoyed by swimmers, bikers, hikers, and dancers. "Exercise exhilaration," a more accurate term, is partially a result of the release of endorphins from the pituitary gland. Vigorous exercise can increase endorphin levels as much as five times.

Aerobic exercise can also help people overcome depression. One reason is the increase in the release of norepinephrine, a deficiency of which has been indicated in depression. Another factor is that the lack of exercise may itself contribute to depression.

Clearly, aerobic exercise works wonders on all three sides of the Holistic Triangle: On the mental/spiritual side it helps you love yourself and experience more joy; on the chemical side it burns calories and releases "feel-good" hormones, such as norepinephrine and endorphin; and on the physical side it builds muscular and cardiovascular fitness. There's no doubt aerobic exercise is an essential element of your Self-Health Program; now it's a matter of choosing which form of aerobics is best for you.

The type of aerobic activity you do, as well as the frequency and duration, initially depends on your current level of fitness. For this reason, four fitness categories are offered: level 1, level 2, level 3, and level 4. When you choose your level, be realistic and honest. Don't feel bad if you're in level 4; you can probably work your way up to level 2 at least by the end of the Self-Health Program. These levels are not meant to be judgmental; they're only to protect you against overdoing it.

These levels are designated for people within the approximate age range of twenty-two to sixty. If you are older, your level will depend on your health history and how often you exercise. If you have any doubts, choose a level with a higher number to be safe, and start your exercise program slowly and carefully.

Level 1: ideal weight and already involved in a rigorous exercise program on a regular basis

Level 2: ideal to moderate weight and intermittent exercise, fairly active, no major health problems

Level 3: moderate to heavy weight and/or no regular exercise, inactive lifestyle

Level 4: overweight and no exercise and/or preexisting physical condition such as severe arthritis, heart disease, or disabilities

Aerobic Activity Choices

Running: Level 1 only to start. Level 2 can build up to it.

Walking:	All levels; distance and speed will depend on capabilities. Not recommended for those with severe arthritis in hips or knees.
Swimming:	Recommended for all levels; distance and speed will depend on level.
Aerobic Dance/ Step Aerobics:	Levels 1 and 2. Level 3 can build up to it. Not recommended if arthritis or injuries exist.
Biking:	Levels 1 and 2. Level 3 can build up to it.
Racquet sports:	Levels 1 and 2. Level 3 needs to start slowly.

Warning Signs

Whatever your level of fitness, you should have a checkup with a doctor before starting or accelerating your exercise program. The reason for this precaution is that only a professional can determine if you have a hidden heart weakness or other condition. Some of the warning signs of a heart condition are:

—Rapid resting pulse
—Irregular pulse
—Shortness of breath
—Pain or discomfort in the chest, abdomen, back, neck, jaw, or arms (can be referred pain from heart)

Although we need to exercise to keep our hearts healthy, we must be careful not to put too much sudden strain on the cardiovascular system. Following are some of the warning signs to watch out for during exercise.

If you experience any of these signs, or any sharp pain, before or during exercise, stop and have a thorough medical examination before you continue:

• Extremely rapid heart rate
• Irregular heartbeat
• Shortness of breath
• Difficulty breathing
• Dizziness or fainting
• Sudden sharp pain or recurrent pain

Running

Running builds cardiovascular capacity efficiently, burns calories quickly, and is one of the best ways to release endorphins and enjoy the mental benefits of aerobic exercise. But there are some drawbacks to consider.

Running, particularly on asphalt, puts a tremendous strain on the joints. Knee injuries are very common among runners, as are muscle pains, tendinitis, and hip injuries. It's not called jogging for nothing; the movement actually jogs your entire body, over and over again.

Another problem is the stress running puts on your lungs, heart, and circulatory system. The level of exertion means that running is a highly beneficial form of exercise but is risky for people with heart conditions. Since heart conditions may be hidden, you should have a complete cardiovascular examination before you take up running. If you learn that you do have a cardiovascular weakness, walking or swimming is a safer aerobic pursuit.

Running is never an entirely risk-free pursuit, but there are precautions that can reduce the chance of injury:

—Purchase a good pair of running shoes from a store where the staff is knowledgeable about runners' needs.
—Warm up before running with a gentle stretching routine.
—Run on a running track or a dirt trail instead of asphalt.
—Cool down with walking after your run.
—Stretch and take a warm bath after the workout.

Walking

Walking is more than exercise; it is a basic human activity that is meant to be part of our lives. It clears the mind and calms the soul as it nourishes the physical side of the Holistic Triangle. Walking is one of the most natural, gentle, yet beneficial forms of exercise.

A study by the Institute for Aerobics Research found brisk

walking improves the body's oxygen uptake and cardiovascular strength. A minimum of twenty minutes of brisk walking at least three times a week will keep your heart healthier and can help control mildly high blood pressure. Start at half a mile per day, and build up distance and speed gradually.

Wear comfortable clothing and good sneakers or walking shoes for your walks. As you walk, breathe deeply through your nose. Try to think positive, relaxed thoughts; don't dwell on problems. If you let your worries go, you may find creative solutions arise during or after your walk.

Follow a natural stride, with flexibility in the hips and torso. Keep your neck and shoulders relaxed. Keep your arms bent at the elbows, swinging back and forth naturally. After your walk, do some gentle stretches.

Swimming

Swimming is the ultimate holistic exercise: It soothes the spirit, stretches the joints, tones the muscles, and works the cardiovascular system. It is also our only opportunity to escape completely from gravity and experience the natural wonder of buoyancy.

Swimming is the one aerobic exercise that can be recommended to almost anyone. It's a particularly good choice for people with arthritis or the elderly, who may not be able to participate in other aerobic activities.

Even with the gentle art of swimming it's wise to start off slowly if you are at fitness levels 3 or 4. You may want to spend a few sessions simply walking back and forth in the water and stretching in the shallow area. Stretching in the water before and after swimming is also therapeutic for advanced swimmers.

The precautions for swimmers are mostly common sense. First of all, be sure you can swim well if you're going in deep water. Wear goggles to avoid getting chlorine in your eyes. Don't swim underwater for a prolonged period of time. If you're swimming in a natural body of water, such as a lake or ocean, always have someone with you.

Many of us were taught to lift our heads only to one side when doing the crawl. A more symmetrical and balanced form is to alternate lifting your head to both sides. The best workout is provided when you do a variety of strokes, including the breaststroke and the backstroke.

As with running and walking, swimming both stimulates and relaxes the mental/spiritual side. Some people like to combine swimming and meditation by concentrating on a mantra or the rhythm of their breaths. Others simply "go with the flow" and find creative thinking is enhanced during and after the swim.

Dancing

Aerobic dancing enjoyed a great vogue, followed by a backlash because of a high rate of injuries. Most aerobic dancing classes and videos were then modified to reduce the impact and potential for injury.

If you are a fitness level 1 or 2, aerobic dancing can be a good workout, but you need to ascertain that your instructor is well educated about safety. Low-impact classes or videotapes with nonjumping movements are recommended.

Work out only on cushioned health club floors or wooden floors, and wear supportive aerobic sneakers. If you have arthritis or a history of joint injuries, aerobic dancing is not a safe exercise choice.

Many of the same precautions apply to aerobic step classes. Those with a high level of fitness can include step training in their regimen, but this should not be the only aerobic activity.

Social dancing, while it is not as cardiovascular-intensive as aerobic dancing, can be good exercise and very pleasurable. The trick to dancing as exercise is to go out to a dance venue where you can keep moving; a couple of slow dances between dinner and dessert isn't going to work.

Dancing in all its forms, from rock-and-rolling around your room to a Broadway jazz class, is a wonderful way to get exercise and express yourself at the same time. Dancing oxygenates the body, strengthens and limbers the muscles, and releases the emotions. Music provides inspiration and energy as the rhythm echoes the heartbeat.

If you've always wanted to be a dancer, you can be one now, as part of your Holistic Self-Health Program. Just be sure to warm up and stretch out before dancing, and don't do movements that feel forced or unnatural. Whether you dance on your own or in a class, keep breathing, don't judge yourself in the mirror, be playful, and enjoy. Keep moving, vary your motions, and revel in the natural expression of your body.

Trampolines are another fun form of aerobic exercise. Minitrampolines can be purchased for home use and are an excellent way to work out without the stress of impact aerobics.

Biking and Racquet Sports

Outdoor biking is a refreshing activity that allows you to appreciate nature while you strengthen your physical side. However, bike riding on a regular basis is not a safe activity for everybody. If you have arthritis, a history of knee injuries, or back pain, walking or swimming may be a better choice since bike riding can place pressure on the joints and compress the spine.

English racers, which are ridden with the torso almost parallel to the ground, relieve this spinal compression, but you need to be fairly slim and strong to be able to handle this type of bike. If you ride a regular or mountain bike in a sitting-up position, get a spring seat and high handlebars so you can sit with a good lumbar curve.

Stationary bikes can provide solid muscular and cardiovascular conditioning. Be sure to purchase a dual-action bike that works the upper body as well as the legs.

Racquet sports are exciting, social activities that also build cardiovascular fitness. The competition and fast pace of racquet sports can motivate people who get bored easily with other exercise.

The problem with racquet sports, and with golf, is that they work one side of the body more than the other. This can result in asymmetrical muscle development, spinal disk problems, and postural distortion.

If you play these sports, you can compensate by working your body through a range of motion in the other direction to create muscular and spinal balance. For instance, if you play tennis with your right arm, address the imbalance by swinging the racquet in your left arm repeatedly before or after your game.

If you find yourself spending more time picking up the ball rather than playing, consider adding another form of exercise for a more sustained cardiovascular workout.

MUSCULOSKELETAL DEVELOPMENT

The goal of musculoskeletal development is to increase the strength, endurance, and flexibility of the skeletal muscles of the body. Muscular strength is the force the muscle produces in one effort; endurance is the ability to perform repeated muscular contractions in quick succession, and flexibility is the full range of motion.

Everyone knows muscular development will make you stronger and more physically attractive. But you may not be aware of the deeper effects of muscular strength and why it is so necessary.

The "inherent tone of the muscle" is the tone the muscle has in a relaxed, steady state. This inherent tone exerts pressure on the bone, which stimulates the bone to absorb calcium, which maintains the strength of the bone itself. Good muscle tone is needed to exert sufficient pressure on the bones, to keep them strong and reduce the likelihood of osteoporosis.

Muscle tone also affects blood circulation. For example, when the calf muscles are flaccid, they don't exert enough pressure on the veins. This can lead to varicose veins and phlebitis and, in extreme cases, the formation of blood clots, which can result in strokes.

The abdominal muscles are the weakest muscle group for most people. The abdominal muscles are responsible for taking the weight off the upper body and into the pelvis. When the abdominals are weak, it puts the burden of support on the lower back and often leads to lower back pain. Most people with lower back pain need to strengthen their abs.

Healthy development of the chest muscles is a prerequisite for efficient chest expansion and oxygen intake. Back muscles, since they are constantly working against gravity, are usually too tight rather than too weak and need to be put through a range of motion. Otherwise the constriction can result in lumbago: being painfully stuck in a contracted position. Neck and shoulder muscles are also frequently tight, resulting in neck pain and tension headaches.

The goal of musculoskeletal exercise is to increase the size of the muscle so it becomes stronger and more capable of doing its job without strain. When a muscle is well developed, the burden is distributed and the muscle is under less stress. There is greater blood flow and less muscle contraction and chance of pain and imbalance.

Just as everyone's Holistic Triangle is different, so everyone has a different state of muscular development, depending on age, frequency of exercise, type of job, and genetics. You'll want to work all your muscle groups, but there are certain areas on which you may need to concentrate.

A self-examination of your muscles can give you guidance on which ones you need to develop. Start by flexing your right calf as strongly as you can, then pressing your index finger into the center of the muscle. If your finger sinks in only a quarter of an inch or less, the tone in the muscle is quite good. If your finger sinks in more than half an inch, the muscle is weak.

Try the same flexion and finger pressure test with your thigh, abdominal, back, chest and arm muscles. Take note of the results so you can emphasize exercises to build these muscles.

Another indicator of health involves the triceps muscles in the back of the arms. Most everyday work is done by the biceps (the front arm muscles), while the triceps are often neglected. But since the triceps are utilized in most aerobic exercises, they are a barometer of cardiovascular health. Weak, flaccid triceps indicate you're not doing enough for your heart.

Another aspect of muscular development to consider is symmetry. Most adults have asymmetrical muscles, which can lead to pressure on the spinal disks and joints and ensuing pain.

Ask a friend or your spouse, workout partner, or doctor to help you inspect your muscular symmetry. Lie flat on the floor, put your arms behind your head, and lift your chin and chest off the floor at a forty-five-degree angle. The person who is studying you can usually supply information about which side has greater muscular development. Then you can do repetitions of exercises on the underdeveloped side to improve symmetry.

When you start your musculoskeletal exercise program, begin slowly and gently. Consistency—doing the exercise three times each week—is more desirable than doing a great number of repetitions infrequently. The number of reps will vary greatly depending on the current state of the physical side of your Holistic Triangle. Keep a record of the number when you start, and gradually increase the repetitions as you strengthen your physical side.

See page 211 for a series of basic musculoskeletal development exercises.

STRETCHING

Stretching is essential for keeping the spine aligned, the muscles fluid, and the joints lubricated. Stretching should be done every day, by everybody.

Animals stretch; it's instinctive and natural. But since we human beings spend so much time in unnatural positions, we have to be careful not to overstretch or to stretch too suddenly.

As you stretch, breathe deeply into your diaphragm. Think of breathing into the stretch; don't pull, bounce, or force. Be very, very gentle and aware. We all have structural and age limitations and need to listen to our bodies.

Try to focus on relaxing, positive thoughts as you stretch. This can be a nice time to do affirmations or active meditation.

Do your stretching on a padded surface—an exercise mat or a thick carpet. If you have the opportunity to stretch on a picnic blanket on the grass or a towel on the beach, that's an added pleasure.

See page 215 for a stretching sequence which provides overall flexibility.

YOGA

Most stretching exercises are based on yoga movements. The deep breathing used in meditation and relaxation is also called yoga breathing. And the Total Body Relaxation on page 218 is often done in yoga classes.

Yoga is stretching, strengthening, breathing, relaxing, meditating, and much more. It is an ancient art and science with a profound spiritual base. Much of the theory and practice of modern holism is based on ancient yogic teachings.

Yoga, born in India thousands of years ago, is probably the original Self-Health Program. It offers a wealth of wisdom that is as valuable today as it was a millennium ago. Yoga encompasses an incredible variety of practices for development of the mind/body and is practiced all over the world, in a multitude of forms.

The term "yoga" is based on the Sanskrit word which means "union" or "joining." This refers to the joining of the physical, mental, and spiritual components and, on a higher level, the joining of human beings and God.

This section on yoga appears in the "Physical Side of Your Holistic Triangle" chapter because many Westerners focus on the poses and breathing practices of yoga. But yoga could also be included in the mental/spiritual chapter since spirituality is a primary element. Some forms of yoga, in fact, focus entirely on spiritual development, meditation, philosophy, moral living, and helping others.

Yoga also influences the chemical side of the Triangle since it advocates the basic health food principles: vegetarianism; sobriety; avoiding dairy products and caffeine; eating wholesome raw foods.

Hatha yoga is the most familiar form of yoga in the United

States. Ideally, hatha yoga is the path to a greater realization of God through mental and physical control. This is achieved through meditation, breathing exercises, and asanas (also called poses or postures).

The asanas move the body through a full range of motions and affect all the body systems: muscular, nervous, digestive, respiratory, elimination, and endocrine. The physical benefits of yoga, which may have been intuitive to its originators, have now been scientifically proved in many studies.

Yoga is open to all ages and levels of fitness, although the practice of asanas and breathing exercises will vary widely according to abilities. What's wonderful about yoga is that you can start at any time and continue practicing for the rest of your life. Many people, including one of the authors of this book, Anita Bell, find yoga a lifelong source of renewal, strength, comfort, and inspiration.

You can begin to learn about yoga through reading and videotapes at home, but at some point you'll want to seek out a teacher. Yoga is taught everywhere from yoga centers to Y's to health clubs.

Wherever you study, ask about the teacher's accreditation and experience. Look for a teacher who is compassionate, communicative, and inspiring. Some people prefer to learn from yogis and yoginis who live in ashrams and dedicate their lives to yoga. But there are also many excellent teachers who lead secular lives and can relate well to the needs of beginning students. Teachers should be flexible in mind and body, be careful to teach correctly and help students avoid injury, and exhibit love of yoga and love of their students.

DEEP BREATHING

Deep breathing (also called yoga breathing or diaphragmatic breathing) increases oxygen intake, a primary goal on the physical side of the Holistic Triangle. It is also useful as a tool for evoking relaxation, another essential nutrient on the physical side.

Look at a baby breathing, or watch someone in a relaxed state of sleep. His or her abdomen gently expands on the inhalation and contracts on the exhalation. This is deep breathing. It is the most revitalizing form of breathing because it increases blood flow to all the organs and stimulates peristaltic function.

This type of breathing is called diaphragmatic because the lungs rest on the diaphragm, the muscle that separates the chest cavity from the abdomen. To fill the lungs completely, the diaphragm needs to lower so that there will be space for lung expansion. In deep breathing, the abdomen expands with each breath, and the diaphragm lowers and allows the lower lung to fill up with oxygen.

If you are a shallow breather, deep breathing can initially result in hyperventilation, dizziness, anxiety, or nausea. You may have to begin by practicing only four or five deep breaths several times a day for a week or two to become accustomed to this greater oxygen supply.

To experience deep breathing, lie down on your bed or the floor. Put your hands on your abdomen. Remember this maxim: The nose is for breathing; the mouth is for eating.

Exhale completely. Close your mouth, and inhale slowly through your nose, filling your abdomen with breath. You should feel your belly rise under your fingers. Continue to inhale, filling up your rib cage, then your chest. Exhale through your nose as slowly and completely as possible. Practice this several more times.

There is a Sufi saying: "Breathing being the secret of all being, it is the most important of all things." Breath is considered the primary link between mind and body in yoga and other holistic traditions. Modern science confirms this ancient wisdom.

The rhythm of the breath affects the right vagus nerve, which controls the sympathetic nervous system. The sympathetic nervous system regulates the excretion of adrenaline and other hormones. Fear, anger, and sorrow all bring uneven patterns to the breath and arouse the sympathetic nervous system.

The best way to learn the effects of deep breathing is to try it out in different situations. When you are concentrating on complex work, check your breathing. Are you breathing deeply through your nose? It will give you greater concentration and more energy and release useless tension.

The next time you get agitated, notice how you're breathing. Then exhale completely, and begin slowly, very slowly, to fill up your abdomen, your rib cage, and then your chest. You'll find this is an amazing calming agent—nature's tranquilizer. It's nearly impossible to be a nervous wreck when you're doing deep abdominal breathing.

A very simple relaxation exercise utilizes deep breathing: Inhale for a count of eight; hold for a count of four; then exhale for a count of eight. When you are comfortable with this ratio, you can try another pattern: Inhale for eight; hold for four; exhale for twelve counts. You can also create your own rhythm, always exhaling at least as long as you inhale. Counting your breaths clears your mind and is a form of relaxation you can practice anywhere.

THE STRESS REACTION

In reaction to stress the body goes into a reactive state, readying itself for a survival response. This is called the fight or flight response and can include these changes:

- Heartbeat increases.
- Blood pressure goes up.
- Breathing becomes rapid and shallow.
- Blood sugar level rises.
- Senses are heightened.
- Muscles tense for movement or protective actions.
- Blood flow to the digestive organs is constricted.
- Blood flow to the brain and major muscles increases.
- Body perspires to cool itself.

These reactions were mandatory for survival in the days when people needed to fight or flee in response to a threat. They could club a wild boar or run from invading tribes and physically utilize those instinctual responses.

Nowadays, however, most of the threats we face are not of a physical nature, and there is no physical release for our stress response. When your boss is critical, you can't work off the muscle tension by beating him or her over the head with a large stick. When someone cuts in front of you on the freeway, you can't suddenly run through the woods to work off the increased heart rate and muscle tension. Instead the biochemical reaction continues for a prolonged period, resulting in wear and tear on the body's response systems.

Dr. Hans Selye, who was one of the world's leading researchers on the effects of stress, discovered that when the brain perceives stress, it automatically sends a message to the hypothalamus, which then sends impulses to the pituitary gland, which releases hormones to stimulate other glands, such as the adrenals. If this stress response continues, the presence of these stress-response hormones begins to wear down the immunological system, and the body becomes more susceptible to disease.

CONSCIOUS RELAXATION

By consciously evoking relaxation, you can counteract some of the effects of stress. *Conscious* relaxation is different from relaxing by watching TV, reading, or even napping. Conscious relaxation methods include meditation, progressive relaxation, deep breathing, yoga, and biofeedback. They decrease the activity of the sympathetic nervous system and release muscle tension, lower blood pressure, and slow the heart and breathing rates.

Dr. Herbert Benson, a cardiologist who is a leading researcher and writer in the field of psychoneuroimmunology, termed this phenomenon the relaxation response. His best-selling book of this name offers simple ways to elicit this response.

Research has proved that conscious relaxation has many dramatic physiological effects. A study of 150 employees of the New York Telephone Company revealed that those who practiced relaxation had less anxiety, high blood pressure, and insomnia five months after they started. Those who practiced relaxation techniques also had more success in overcoming smoking, drinking alcohol, and overeating habits. Other studies have indicated that relaxation is a major tool in alleviating chronic pain from backache, headache, or such diseases as cancer.

Healing Moments, meditation, and deep breathing are basic relaxation methods you can use. Page 218 offers a Total Body Relaxation sequence, which you can either memorize or read onto a cassette to create your own customized relaxation tape.

BATHING

Water is more than required nourishment on the chemical side of the Triangle; it is also a healing tool on the physical and mental/spiritual sides. Bathing has been used for soothing and healing as well as cleaning the body for thousands of years.

Using hot and cold water in combination can be highly therapeutic. Hot water increases surface circulation, dilates pores, increases elimination through the skin, and helps the muscles to relax. Cold water stimulates the circulation while it contracts the blood vessels and pores of the skin. Bathing is also one of our few opportunities to escape the weight of gravity and the burden it places on our muscles and bones.

On the mental/spiritual side, hydrotherapy gives us a chance to evoke the feeling of being inside the womb. Since we come from water and we're partly composed of water, being in this element relaxes the mind along with the muscles.

See page 219 for a hydrotherapeutic Bathing Ritual that provides spiritual as well as physical nourishment.

SLEEPING

Sufficient sleep is part of your fundamental nourishment on the physical side of your Holistic Triangle. Remember: *Rest* is the greatest *rest*orer of health. No matter how busy you are, try to show your love for yourself by getting enough sleep.

How much sleep is enough is highly personal. Six to eight hours' sleep is the normal range for optimal functioning, but it's variable. Listen to your body, and give it what it needs. However, if you feel you habitually need more than eight hours' sleep a night, this may indicate you need to eat a healthier diet, take more supplements, do more exercise, and/or address feelings of depression.

If you have insomnia, avoid taking sleeping pills, which can be addictive and lead to a host of serious side effects. Instead you can utilize these safe, natural techniques for overcoming sleeplessness:

—Eliminate caffeine, sugar, nicotine, and meat from your diet.
—Eat early, light dinners; then have a small snack two hours before bedtime.
—Get vigorous exercise during the day.
—Get out in the morning daylight (this does not have to be direct sunlight) to adjust your inner clock.
—Go to sleep and get up at approximately the same time every day of the week.
—Do gentle stretches, followed by the Total Body Relaxation sequence, directly before going to bed.
—If your thoughts keep you awake, try a simple meditation by focusing on the word "one" as you exhale. You can also do relaxation practices in bed.
—Reserve your bed for only sleeping (and sex); don't read, eat, or watch TV in bed. Let your mind associate bed with rest.
—Making love and masturbating can help you get to sleep if you are comfortable with your partner and your own sexuality.

How you sleep as well as how much is a consideration on the physical side of the Triangle. Use only one pillow, not too thick, to avoid neck compression. Sleep on your side or on your back, but never on your stomach. Stomach sleeping causes uneven twisting of the cervical vertebrae, which can put the whole spine out of alignment and add pressure to the lower back. When you rise out of bed, turn on your side first and use your hands to push up to a sitting position.

POSTURE

It's ironic that in elementary school, where we're supposed to learn good habits, we learn bad posture. Despite the admonitions of stern teachers to sit up straight, school desks and chairs promote poor postural habits. We learn to slouch in our uncomfortable chairs and look down at our reading and writing. These habits continue into adulthood and are exacerbated by the office environment. The result is frequent lower back pain, neck pain, and headaches.

Lisa, a thirty-two-year-old public relations writer, came to the Holistic Health Force complaining of neck pain and tension headaches. She had a very common distortion pattern: a developing dowager's hump and loss of cervical (neck) curve. Looking at Lisa, you probably wouldn't notice anything was wrong since a slightly forward curve of the neck is such a common trait. But it was enough to cause Lisa neck pain, reduced blood supply to her head, and recurrent headaches.

Lisa was given chiropractic adjustments in our office and muscle work to rehabilitate the supportive elements. However, the principal component of her treatment program was the work she did on her own.

Lisa learned to sleep on her back instead of her stomach and to use a cervical pillow. She started the day with the Bathing Ritual, which was a great relief for her neck. An exercise program of swimming, yoga, and musculoskeletal exercises gave her better alignment, greater strength, and more energy.

At the office Lisa adjusted her computer screen to eye level so she didn't have to look down. She invested in an ergonomic chair and had it delivered to her office. Coffee breaks became stretching breaks. She stopped cramming the phone between her ear and shoulder and held it in her hand, with her head up.

Paying attention to the physical side of her Triangle relieved

THE SKELETAL SYSTEM

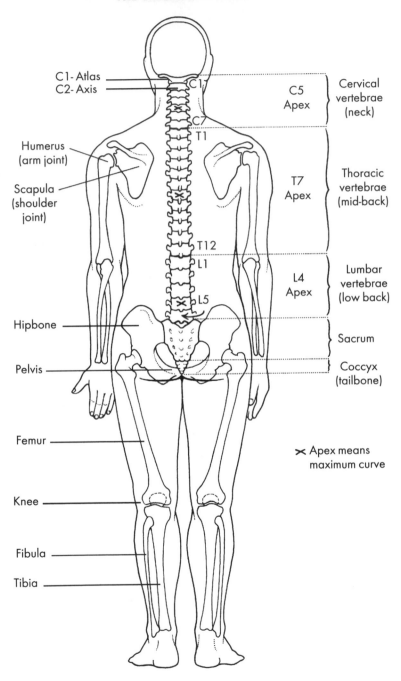

C1- Atlas
C2- Axis

C1
C5
Apex

Cervical
vertebrae
(neck)

Humerus
(arm joint)

C7
T1

Scapula
(shoulder
joint)

T7
Apex

Thoracic
vertebrae
(mid-back)

T12
L1

Hipbone

L4
Apex

L5

Lumbar
vertebrae
(low back)

Pelvis

Sacrum

Coccyx
(tailbone)

Femur

✕ Apex means
maximum curve

Knee

Fibula

Tibia

GOOD POSTURE REFLECTS GOOD HEALTH

Gravitational Forces

Gravitational Forces

UNHEALTHY POSTURE

HEALTHY POSTURE

a. Fatigue and negative thinking

a. Energy and positive thinking

b. Restricted neck, loss of normal curve*

b. Flexible neck with natural curve

c. Rounded, weak shoulders

c. Strong, erect shoulders, normal curve

d. Rigid low back, flattened curve*

d. Flexibility and normal forward curve

e. Reduced pelvic angle with compressed organs

e. Normal pelvic angle with relaxed internal organs

f. Flat feet and poor ankle alignment

f. Good arch (or arch support) and proper ankle alignment

*Results in compressed spinal disks

Note: Poor posture: Center of balance is off

Good posture: Body is balanced and well aligned

Lisa's neck pain and headaches. As a bonus, her improved posture and physical development made her look taller, trimmer, and more attractive.

When working on your posture, remember, a healthy spine is *not* a straight spine. The admonition "Sit up straight" is misleading. The correct goal is to support your spine with strong muscles and to sit or stand with the natural curvature of your spine in place. The illustration on page 93 will give you a visual sense of balanced curvature.

Here are some ways you can nurture your physical side by developing better postural habits:

- Sit tall. Maintain the natural curve in your lower back as you sit; don't slump. Imagine a puppet string pulling you up from the top of your head. Keep your spine long and your gaze ahead, not down.
- Don't cross your legs. Leg crossing causes poor circulation in the legs and vulnerability to varicose veins and phlebitis. It also reverses the normal lumbar lordosis (forward curve) of the lower back and compresses the spinal disks and lower back muscles.
- Work in a healthy chair, even if you need to buy it yourself and have it delivered to your workplace. Get an ergonomically designed desk chair or a kneeling chair that will facilitate good posture.
- Your seat height should allow you to keep your feet flat on the floor and your knees level with or slightly higher than your hips. If you're short, you may need to place something under your feet to achieve this posture. (This rule does not apply to kneeling chairs, which place the knees lower than the hips in a kneeling position.)
- Position your computer screen at eye level. Get a standing clipboard or reading stand so you don't need to peer down at papers. The idea is to look down as little as possible.
- Whenever you read, hold the material up to eye level or use a reading stand; don't look down. If you wear bifocals, hold the reading material slightly below eye level so you can read

through the bottom of your glasses while still maintaining your natural neck curve.

- Holding the telephone between your ear and your shoulder is a recipe for neck pain. Hold the phone with your hand, and keep your head erect. If you often write or type when you're on the phone, purchase a telephone headset to free your hands.
- Stand tall, with your head up, weight balanced on both legs, and spine lengthened. However, you don't want to hyperextend your lower back; maintain the natural curve.
- Look ahead when you walk, not down.
- When carrying heavy packages, hold them close to your body in both arms.
- Squat when you need to lift something; don't bend from the waist.
- If you carry a pocketbook, try to lighten it and take only what's necessary. Wear the strap diagonally across your chest rather than on your shoulder, and alternate sides. Consider using a lightweight backpack instead of a shoulder bag.
- Avoid high heels, which compress the lower back and torture the feet. If you stand tall and exercise frequently, you'll look terrific without heels. Remember, improving your posture results in instant figure enhancement.
- Even with excellent posture, remaining in one position for a long period of time is unnatural and unhealthy. Human beings are meant to be dynamic. Get up, stretch, and walk around the room as often as possible.

SECONDARY FORMS OF PHYSICAL NOURISHMENT

The secondary forms of nourishment on the physical side of the Holistic Triangle are those that are provided by natural health professionals, such as chiropractors, massage therapists, physical therapists, acupuncturists, naturopaths, nutritionists, homeopathic doctors, and others.

One of the ways you can show yourself love is to spend the time and money necessary to get appropriate professional care. Visits to holistic practitioners can be costly, but they serve as a form of health insurance. In many cases, reasonable natural health care has helped people avoid devastatingly expensive surgery.

David, a commercial artist, came to the Holistic Health Force in a last-ditch effort for a second opinion before undergoing back surgery. He had severe sciatica that was no longer relieved by the painkillers his doctor had prescribed. His doctor recommended disk surgery, but as a freelancer with no health insurance David was worried this would wipe him out financially.

A holistic rehabilitation program consisting of chiropractic care, therapeutic exercise, supplementation, and a change of postural habits afforded David pain relief and corrected the imbalance that was causing him pain. He didn't have to submit to surgery, and he stopped taking painkillers. Best of all, he has been able to maintain a healthy back by following his own Holistic Self-Health Program rules and visiting the office only three or four times a year.

Mabel, an eighty-two-year-old woman, was depressed when her doctor told her she had to undergo surgery to remove her painfully inflamed varicose veins. She was afraid of hospitals and believed surgery would be a strain she might not survive.

A holistic program of therapeutic exercise, physiotherapy to strengthen her calf muscles, and chiropractic treatment, combined with weight loss from a customized diet, rendered the surgery unnecessary. Mabel also elevated the foot of her bed and started wearing support panty hose to help her condition.

Within two months Mabel was able to resume her part-time cooking job and activities with her church group. Because of her age, she needs biweekly visits to our office to prevent her condition from deteriorating. But this continuing care is certainly less expensive and invasive than surgery.

These case studies from the Holistic Health Force are a microcosm of the findings of many research studies. AV Med, the largest health maintenance organization (HMO) in the southwestern United States, sent one hundred of its medically unresponsive patients to a chiropractor. Within three weeks 86 percent of these patients had their ailments corrected, and the twelve who had been previously diagnosed as needing disk surgery had their conditions corrected. This saved AV Med approximately $250,000 in surgery costs.

A study of workers' compensation records of more than three thousand cases in Utah found that chiropractic outperformed medicine by a ten-to-one margin in compensation costs. Overseas a study by the Italian government of seventeen thousand patients showed that chiropractic care reduced hospitalization by 87.6 percent and work loss by 75.5 percent.

According to a Rand Corporation study, one fourth of all days spent in the hospital, one fourth of all procedures, and two fifths of medications are unnecessary. One way you can avoid becoming a statistic is to seek out drug-free, noninvasive health care treatments.

There are many different holistic healing therapies, each with its unique strengths. On page 222 you'll find a brief introduction to some of these alternatives. Please keep in mind that these therapies are multifaceted, and you can find whole books devoted to most of them. You may want to support your physical side with mental nourishment by reading in-depth studies of the modalities that interest you.

PART TWO

THE HOLISTIC
SELF-HEALTH
PROGRAM

CHAPTER 5

Ready, Set, Go: Starting Your Self-Health Program

The Three-Month Holistic Self-Health Program is a framework for nourishing the mental/spiritual, chemical, and physical sides of your Holistic Triangle. It will help you systematically utilize the techniques introduced in the previous chapters and mobilize your healing force and energy.

For thousands of years people have searched for the Fountain of Youth. If youth can be equated with feeling young, energetic, limber, strong, and full of hope and optimism, then the Holistic Self-Health Program is an attainable fountain. If you stay with the program, by the end of three months you'll find yourself revitalized, looking and feeling fresher. And if you adopt the principles of the program into your permanent lifestyle, it will help you maintain your vigor and health into your later years.

A three-month span is used for the program because this is the amount of time in which many conditions heal. Three months is a typical period for both the innate self-healing mechanisms of the body and professional treatment programs. In my clinical experience, three months is also the average time it takes many patients to make serious changes in their lifestyles and adopt holistic habits. Of course, the period in which people heal and change is as individual as their Holistic Triangles, and many patients respond in less time, while others take longer.

Before you embark on the Self-Health Program, please understand this is a process, not a pass/fail course. The program is a series of steps and goals, a journey toward health. The ultimate goal is to keep loving yourself to wellness by nourishing your Holistic Triangle as much as you can.

The greatest result you can achieve is to keep trying. If your resolve falters, respond with love and forgiveness instead of berating yourself. Pick yourself up and carry on with the program as best you can.

Like any other endeavor that yields a high-quality result, the Self-Health Program is not easy. Accomplishment is directly proportional to the amount of work you put into the program. However, you'll quickly realize this is the type of work that brings deep satisfaction and pleasure.

Think of gardening, which is hard work that millions of people love. Gardeners begin by preparing the soil and planting the seeds. They weed and water the garden, and with nature's help, it blossoms, bringing a great deal of joy to the cultivator. With the Self-Health Program your hard work and nature's assistance will result in the flowering of your body and spirit.

KEEP THE MOMENTUM GOING

Depending on the present state of your Holistic Triangle and your level of discipline and resolve, you may or may not be able to accomplish all the steps of the program in the three-month period. If this happens, it's critical not to get bogged down. Focus on another side of your Triangle until you've gained the strength to deal with the more difficult area.

For example, if you simply can't give up sugar, set that goal aside for a week, and do an activity on the physical side that will give you a sense of accomplishment: Swim ten extra laps or walk that extra mile. When you've achieved a new level on one side of your Triangle, you may find it gives you confidence and determination to get through the "stuck" area.

If you find it too difficult to accomplish the major goals during your first effort, you can start the process again and reembark on the Self-Health Program for a second or third time. During these repeat cycles of the program, goals that may have seemed too difficult the first time should become more manageable. The more obstacles you work through, the more self-empowerment you'll gain. Instead of the downward spiral, you'll be swept up in a current of positive change.

IT'S NEVER TOO LATE TO CHANGE

When I explain the Holistic Self-Health Program to patients, some of them voice this initial response: "But it's too late for me to change now, Doc."

If this is your attitude, you need to realize that you're going to change whether you want to or not. Life is a process of change; it's inevitable. You have a choice: You can take control of your health and change for the better, or you can avoid responsibility and change for the worse.

Douglas, age sixty, was fifty pounds overweight and had high blood pressure. For years his medical doctor and his wife had urged him to diet and exercise, but he preferred to take his hypertensive medication and continue with his unhealthy lifestyle. It wasn't until he started getting severe headaches as a side effect of the medication that he was motivated to change.

Douglas started by eliminating sugar from his diet and was encouraged by the benefits he felt in a few weeks. This provided the positive reinforcement he needed to start exercising and reducing his intake of other toxins.

Years of ingrained habits were difficult to change, however, and by the end of three months Douglas still consumed too much red meat and beer, was erratic in his exercise program, and hadn't managed a juice fast. He had lost fifteen pounds, and his blood pressure was lower, although not normal. But the progress he had made encouraged him to start on another round of his Self-Health Program.

During the next cycle Douglas finally broke his red meat habit and actually started to look forward to his daily health walks. His wife went on a juice fast at the same time he did, and that made it easier for him to get through it.

By the end of the second three months, Douglas had lost an additional twenty pounds and reduced his blood pressure to the point where medication was no longer required. He felt full of vim and vigor, and his family joked that he looked better than his thirty-eight-year-old son. Douglas was living proof that it's never too late to change.

MAKING TIME FOR YOURSELF

Another negative response I often hear from patients about the program is: "I'm too busy; I don't have time." This is certainly a valid concern. Lack of time is a major area of stress in today's world and is connected with the ever-present worry about money. But we need to find balance; we can't always put work ahead of health.

"Health is wealth" is a cliché because it happens to be true. Not only is it difficult to enjoy money if you're unhealthy, but it's also hard to earn it. If you don't take time out for now for self-nourishment, in the future your earning capacity may be disrupted by premature illness that prevents you from working at all.

No matter what your responsibilities, you deserve and require a certain amount of time for yourself. And this time, if it is limited, needs to be spent in the most positive way possible: nourishing your Holistic Triangle. The greatest gift you can give yourself is time.

Li, a forty-five-year-old teacher, came in complaining of neck and shoulder pain. An examination found that she had the beginnings of arthritis and a reversal of the normal neck curve (cervical lordosis). This is a common condition that results from neck stress, looking down, and using too many pillows.

After three weeks of chiropractic adjustments to align the vertebrae, ultrasound to break down scar tissue, and electrical therapy to reduce inflammation, her pain was gone. She then decided she didn't have time to go on the Holistic Self-Health Program; she was too busy with her high school teaching position and additional evening job teaching English as a second language to adults.

A few months later she returned to the office with a recurrence of neck and shoulder pain, this time more severe. Now she was ready to embark on the exercise part of the program, but she still didn't know why she should bother changing her diet if the pain was in her neck.

Then we discussed the results of a Nutriscan test of her blood. (Nutriscan tests are a comprehensive chemical analysis of the blood to determine the level of vitamins and minerals.) This test showed she lacked beta-carotene and other nutrients that were indicated for the prevention of cancer. Since Li had already had a melanoma removed from her back, she was very concerned about cancer, and this news motivated her to work on the chemical side of her Triangle as well as the physical side.

Li realized she needed to drop one of the night classes to make time to exercise regularly, practice relaxation, and prepare fresh meals for herself. Once she began to apply her high level of discipline and determination to loving herself, she made rapid progress in building up her Triangle.

HINTS FOR BUSY PEOPLE

When you first read through the program, it may sound like a lot to do, and you may worry that you won't find the time. Please realize that in most cases it's a matter of replacing present habits with more nourishing activities, and you will not need to "make" a lot of time.

Here are tips on how to manage the program in a "timely" fashion:

Mental/Spiritual Side

- Practice Healing Moments as a quick and effective way to nourish your spiritual side.
- Practice deep breathing in the car, while waiting on lines, and whenever else you can think of it.
- Affirmations can be done during any spare moments. Another idea: Every time you start worrying, try to replace the worrisome thoughts with affirmations.
- Do a relaxation or visualization session instead of watching a half hour sitcom.
- For the three months of the program consider giving up reading your daily newspaper and spend the time reading more uplifting material.
- Replace your daily shower with the Bathing Ritual. Set your alarm clock fifteen minutes earlier so you have time for the Healing Moments and exercises in the bathtub. The sense of well-being will more than compensate for a little less sleep.

Chemical Side

- Raw, natural foods are quicker and easier to prepare than many typical American meals. Instead of spending time on elaborate recipes, stick to simple, nourishing foods that give you strength for the rest of your activities.
- You can prepare raw juices on weekends and freeze them to use during the week. (They are most nourishing when fresh, but if you're extremely pressed for time on workdays, this is an alternative.)
- Set your supplements out in the kitchen, and establish a habit of taking them before meals; this takes very little time.

- Eliminating toxins—one of the most important steps in the program—will give you more energy and time for the rest.

Physical Side

- Exercise with friends, partners, or children so it can be a social as well as physical time.
- Cut down on shopping and watching TV during the three months of the program so you have more time for physically active pursuits.
- If you have a baby, use his or her nap time as your exercise time. Even when you're exhausted, this is likely to give you more energy for the rest of the day.

*A note of caution: It is *recommended that you do not go on the Self-Health Program during pregnancy.*

SHARE THE PROGRAM WITH IMPORTANT PEOPLE IN YOUR LIFE

Being involved in the program will mean certain changes in your eating habits, exercise routine, and other aspects of your lifestyle. It's helpful to explain to your family, partner, close friends, or relatives what you are trying to achieve so they won't stand in the way of your goals.

You may want to show them this book and have them leaf through it. Or you can describe in your own words your desire to enhance your well-being through the program. Present the information in whatever way you think is appropriate, but try not to preach or drown other people in ideas.

Most people are resistant to change, and you may encounter naysaying and skepticism. Even the people who love you dearly and wish you well may disappoint you with their lack of support. Try not to take it too personally. Everyone is at a different stage of mental/spiritual development, and many intelligent and well-meaning people are still not open to new ideas about health. You can inform people, but you can't force anyone to listen, and proselytizing tends to strengthen resistance.

The very best way you can convince other people of the validity of the Self-Health Program is to set an example. Let them see how it benefits you, and it may open their minds. Ultimately, however, you're responsible only for yourself; you cannot create total well-being for anyone else.

THE BUDDY SYSTEM

If your spouse, partner, friend, relative, or colleague is genuinely interested in the Holistic Self-Health Program, you may want to invite her or him to be your "buddy" throughout the process. The buddy system is often used in self-help programs and can be helpful and fun.

Let your potential buddy read this book and decide if he or she would like to go on the program with you. If you use the buddy system, these are some of the ways you can help each other:

—Share books on holistic topics and discuss ideas.
—Go to lectures, seminars, and workshops together to strengthen your mental/spiritual sides.
—Practice meditation and relaxation techniques together, and discuss which practices you find most nourishing.
—Share cookbooks and natural food recipes.
—Prepare and eat healthy meals together.
—Call on each other for verbal support when you are eliminating toxins.
—Go on a raw-juice fast at the same time.
—Embark on an exercise program together.
—Work out together on a regular basis to keep the momentum going.
—Openly discuss procrastination, resistance, and setbacks you encounter during the program.
—Give each other affirmation and recognition of your efforts and progress.

—Celebrate your progress with a special treat, such as a professional massage, a weekend in the country, or a party with lots of delicious natural food.

As delightful as it is to have a buddy during the Self-Health Program, it is not necessary. You can be your own buddy and give yourself encouragement and support through self-nourishing practices. The program is designed to be an independent effort, although you will need an initial checkup from a health care professional before starting.

CHOOSING A NATURAL DOCTOR

Before you begin the Self-Health Program, it is required, as mentioned earlier, that you have a doctor give you an examination to determine that there are no hidden conditions that you need to consider. I recommend a complete physical checkup that includes an assessment of health history, height, weight, blood pressure, a cardiovascular examination (including an EKG if you are over forty-five), a musculoskeletal examination, and a blood work-up.

The comprehensive chemical profile of your blood will test the size, type, and differentiation of red and white blood cells and help identify such underlying conditions as hypoglycemia, anemia, thyroid malfunctions, vascular disease, and deficiencies. These tests should be performed by a qualified doctor who will take the time to communicate with you about the results.

The Three-Month Holistic Self-Health program is primarily a series of self-help activities. However, in addition to the mandatory checkup before starting the program, it is helpful to maintain contact with a health care professional who can provide supervision and encouragement during the process. Before starting the program, you may want to seek out a holistic practitioner from one of the following disciplines:

Natural chiropractic physician (D.C.): This person should be knowledgeable about nutrition and exercise, as well as physiology, and believe in helping patients achieve independent good health.

Natural medical doctor or physician (M.D.): Some medical doctors are now embracing a more holistic approach. If you work with a holistic medical doctor, ascertain that he or she is committed to the natural approach and will not encourage drug therapy or surgical intervention.

Natural Doctor of Osteopathy (D.O.): Osteopathic physicians provide comprehensive medical care, with particular attention to joints, bones, muscles, and nerves. D.O.'s can prescribe drugs or surgery, so if you are working with one, you need to establish clearly if she or he is dedicated to natural healing. Also inquire about the D.O.'s experience with nutritional counseling.

Naturopathic physician: Naturopaths utilize a wide variety of holistic modalities that may complement the Self-Health Program. However, since they are licensed only in seven states at this time, qualified naturopaths can be difficult to locate.

Personal recommendations from friends, family, and colleagues are helpful in finding a new doctor. If you need to start from scratch, you can look for practitioners who advertise in natural health publications in your area, call professional associations, or even check the phone book. When you don't know anyone who has worked with the practitioner before, however, you need to be especially cautious.

Start with a phone call and ask to speak to the professional directly. He or she should be willing to answer basic questions about training, certification, scope of practice, methods of treatment, and use of tests. The doctor should have a friendly, enthusiastic manner and give you a positive first impression. If you have a gut feeling she or he is wrong for you, either on the phone or during the initial consultation, pay attention to your instincts and look for someone else.

During the initial consultation, assess whether the doctor's fees, insurance arrangements, location, and schedule fit your budget and lifestyle. Take note of the practitioner's human skills, her or his attitude toward holism, and his or her willingness to answer questions.

After the first examination, see if the doctor gives you sufficient information about your current state of health and explains recommendations. If treatment is needed, he or she should outline the timetable (although this can never be absolute), the approximate cost, and the pros and cons of different treatments.

Your health care provider should have excellent professional qualifications, but she or he also needs strong interpersonal skills and qualities. The doctor should be a teacher, who will take the time to talk with you about your present state of health, how your body works, and what you can do for yourself. You should feel his or her genuine interest and compassion. A sense of humor and natural warmth is a plus. Your doctor should treat you as an equal and a partner in your health and not have a condescending attitude.

As holistic health gains in popularity, some doctors may call themselves holistic though they are not truly committed to a natural approach. Therefore, it's necessary to determine that your doctor will not rely on drugs, surgery, or quick fixes but will emphasize and explore a variety of natural remedies. The professional should be dedicated to finding and correcting the root cause of problems, not just covering symptoms. To be considered sincerely holistic, he or she should have a deep belief in the integral connection of the mind, spirit, and body and view you as a whole person, not as a series of symptoms.

A holistic doctor should recognize the essential connection between nutrition and good health and have a background in nutrition. She or he should also be acquainted with therapeutic exercise and relaxation techniques.

It's helpful to have your doctor look at this book, and you should then explain that you would like her or his support during the Holistic Self-Health Program. After your initial comprehensive exam, the practitioner should review the program and let you know if your tests indicate any special precautions should be taken.

THE SELF-HEALTH EVALUATIONS

While clinical tests given by a health care professional are useful, they are limited in scope. Clinical tests are aimed at identifying deficiencies, illnesses, and weaknesses rather than strengths. The following Self-Health Evaluations are designed to clarify both your strong points and weaknesses on all three sides of your Holistic Triangle.

Take the tests now, review the results, and then save them. When you take the tests again at the end of the Three-Month Holistic Self-Health Program, you can chart your progress. This is, of course, just reinforcement since your progress will be evident from the way you feel, think, and look.

No test can define a human being, and the following evaluations cannot present a definitive picture of your infinitely complex self. The goal of these tests is to get you thinking about the state of your Holistic Triangle and what you can do to nourish it. The tests are a learning tool, not a judgment. For this reason, the scores are not separated into categories such as "good, mediocre, awful." The numerical scores are intended to help you compare the relative strengths of each side of your Holistic Triangle and to help you see how you are benefiting from the program when you retake the tests after three months.

Answer the questions to the best of your ability; circle your answers; then add up your score. The higher the score, the stronger you are on this particular side of your Triangle. The lower your score, the more attention you need to pay to nourishing this side.

The Mental/Spiritual Side Evaluation

1. Overall, would you say you give yourself enough unconditional love and acceptance?

   1-No   2-Sometimes, but not usually   3-Yes

2. Do you consider yourself a positive thinker?

   1-No   2-Somewhat   3-Yes

3. How do you rate your level of self-esteem?
   1-Low   2-Medium   3-High

4. How often do you feel fearful?
   1-Often   2-Occasionally   3-Rarely or never

5. How often do you feel guilty?
   1-Often   2-Occasionally   3-Rarely or never

6. How often do you feel depressed?
   1-Often   2-Occasionally   3-Rarely or never

7. How often do you feel anxious?
   1-Often   2-Occasionally   3-Rarely

8. Do you wake up looking forward to your day?
   1-Never or rarely   2-Sometimes   3-Most days

9. Do you enjoy your work?
   1-No or very little   2-Somewhat   3-Very much

10. Do you feel satisfied with spouse or partner?
    1-No or don't have one   2-Somewhat   3-Very much

11. Do you feel satisfied with the quality of your friendships?
    1-No   2-Somewhat   3-Very much

12. Do you do volunteer work, or otherwise help people outside your own family?
    1-Never or rarely   2-Occasionally   3-On a regular basis

13. Do you consider yourself a spiritual person?
    1-No   2-Somewhat   3-Yes

14. Do you engage in religious/spiritual practices?
    1-Never or rarely   2-Occasionally   3-Frequently

15. Do you meditate, do affirmations and visualizations, and/or practice relaxation techniques?
    1-Never or rarely   2-Occasionally   3-Frequently

16. Do you read books on spiritual and/or holistic health topics?
    1-Rarely   2-Occasionally   3-Frequently

17. Do you believe in your innate healing force?

    1-No   2-Not sure   3-Yes

18. Do you believe your mental/spiritual state has a profound effect on your health?

    1-No   2-Not sure   3-Yes

19. What is your level of discipline when it comes to making healthy choices?

    1-Low   2-Medium   3-High

20. Do you believe you have the power substantially to improve your mental and physical well-being?

    1-No   2-Not sure   3-Yes

The Chemical Side Evaluation

Note: Since eating habits vary, try to answer the questions according to your general pattern.

1. How often do you consume sugar?

   1-More than twice a week   2-Once or twice a week   3-Rarely or never

2. How often do you eat white flour products and other refined carbohydrates?

   1-More than twice a week   2-Once or twice a week   3-Rarely or never

3. How often do you eat dairy products?

   1-More than twice a week   2-Once or twice a week   3-Rarely or never

4. How often do you eat meat?

   1-More than twice a week   2-Once or twice a week   3-Rarely or never

5. How often do you consume foods with additives (or added salt)?

   1-More than twice a week   2-Once or twice a week   3-Rarely or never

6. How often do you smoke?

   1-Daily or often   2-Rarely   3-Never

7. How often do you consume caffeine?

   1-Daily or often   2-Rarely   3-Never

8. How many glasses of alcohol, wine, or beer do you have per week?

   1-More than seven   2-Three to five   3-Two or less

9. How often do you take drugs, including recreational drugs, prescriptions, and over-the-counter medications?

   1-One to seven times per week   2-Once a month to several times a year   3 Rarely or never

10. How would you rate your exposure to environmental toxins?

    1-High   2-Average   3-Low

11. How often do you eat vegetables and salads?

    1-A few times a week or less   2-Three to six times a week   3-Every day

12. How often do you eat fruits or drink raw-fruit juices?

    1-A few times a week or less   2-Three to six times a week   3-Every day

13. How often do you eat legumes, nuts, and seeds?

    1-A few times a week or less   2-Three to five times a week   3-Six or more times a week

14. How often do you eat whole grains?

    1-A few times a week or less   2-Three to six times a week   3-Six or more times a week

16. How frequently do you go on a raw-juice fast?

    1-Never   2-Once or twice a year   3-More than twice a year

17. How many glasses of pure water do you drink each day?

    1-Zero to three glasses   2-Four to five glasses   3-More than five glasses

18. Do you have regular bowel movements without straining?
    1-Rarely or never 2-Sometimes 3-Usually

19. Do you eat six small meals, with the largest portion at lunch-time?
    1-Rarely or never 2-Sometimes 3-Usually

20. Do you take vitamin and mineral supplements?
    1-Rarely or never 2-Sometimes 3-Habitually

The Physical Side Evaluation

1. How often do you do aerobic (cardiovascular) exercise?
   1-Less than once a week 2-Once or twice a week 3-Three or more times a week

2. What is the average duration of your aerobic workout?
   1-Less than fifteen minutes 2-Fifteen to thirty minutes 3-Over thirty minutes

3. How long can you do aerobic activity without becoming short of breath?
   1-Don't know, or less than fifteen minutes 2-Fifteen to thirty minutes 3-Over thirty minutes

4. How often do you do musculoskeletal exercise?
   1-Less than once a week 2-Once or twice a week 3-Three or more times a week

5. How many sit-ups (as described in Chapter 5) can you do without feeling neck strain?
   1-Less than five 2-Five to twenty 3-Over twenty

6. How many push-ups can you do while maintaining form? (Women can test with modified push-ups.)
   1-Less than five 2-Five to twenty 3-Over twenty

7. How often do you do limbering and stretching exercises or yoga?
   1-Less than once a week 2-One to four times week 3-More than four times a week

8. Can you touch your toes, keeping your legs straight?
   1-No   2-Yes, with effort   3-Can place palms on floor

9. Can you reach your arms over your shoulders and touch your back between your shoulder blades?
   1-No   2-Yes, with effort   3-Easily

10. According to the criteria on page 75, what is your level of fitness?
    1-Level 3 or 4   2-Level 2   3-Level 1

11. How close is your current weight to your ideal weight?
    1-Want to lose over twenty pounds   2-Want to lose three to twenty pounds   3-Close to or at ideal weight.

12. How would you rate your level of energy?
    1-Low   2-Medium   3-High

13. How often do you practice deep breathing?
    1-Rarely or never   2-Occasionally   3-Often

14. How often do you practice a technique to evoke conscious relaxation?
    1-Rarely or never   2-Occasionally   3-Often

15. How often do you do the Bathing Ritual?
    1-Rarely or never   2-Occasionally   3-Often

16. In what position do you usually sleep?
    1-On stomach   2-Various positions with two pillows   3-On back or side with one pillow

17. How would you rate your sleep generally?
    1-Poor, not enough, and/or insomnia   2-Adequate, sometimes not enough, or insomnia   3-Good

18. How is your posture while you are working?
    1-Poor   2-Fair   3-Good

19. Do you sit with your legs crossed?
    1-Often   2-Occasionally   3-Rarely or never

20. How often do you see a holistic health practitioner?

    1-Rarely or never   2-Occasionally, usually when in pain
    3-On a regular basis

Your Family Health History

In a notebook or journal, write down the names of your maternal and paternal grandparents, parents, brothers, and sisters. Next to each name, write down any major illnesses the relative had and the cause of death if he or she is deceased.

The purpose of this evaluation is to see what diseases "run in the family." Then you can take extra preventive measures to reduce your chances of developing these illnesses.

Family history does not have to be destiny; it can be a useful tool in loving yourself to health. Although genetics create a predisposition, you can build up immunity by nourishing your Triangle and, in many cases, avoid the illnesses of your ancestors. Continue to note down your own health history.

Your Health History

1. List any diseases you've had in the past.
2. List any injuries and operations you've had.
3. List any episodes of chronic pain or complaints.
4. List all the messages your body has given you recently. Messages can be in the form of pain, discomfort, conditions, diseases, allergies, breathing problems, digestive disorders, and weaknesses. (The term "messages" is used instead of "symptoms" to remind you to pay attention to what they have to say.)

   Next to each message, make a note of the frequency of occurrence and degree of severity.

Message   *Frequency*   *Severity*

Take some time to study the messages your body has given you in the past and the present. It is likely that if you follow through with the Holistic Self-Health Program, in three months you will see a significant change.

SET YOUR STARTING DATE

The final step in preparing for the program is to pick a date to begin it. Try to choose a period when you will not be under any extraordinary demands at work or at home. However, don't wait until a time when you have no stress at all, or you may never get to the program. Remember, you can fit the program into your life by replacing many present activities and habits with more beneficial ones.

Once this date is set, it should be a firm commitment and a top priority. Don't procrastinate or invent rationalizations as to why you should postpone beginning the program. The sooner you start, the sooner you can begin your progress toward total well-being.

CHECKLIST FOR STARTING YOUR HOLISTIC SELF-HEALTH PROGRAM

❑ Make a commitment to create positive change and spend time on more nourishing activities.

❑ Explain to your family and close friends that you will be on a special program. Enlist a buddy for support if you wish.

❑ Select a holistic doctor who communicates well and treats you as a partner.

❑ Have a comprehensive professional examination to determine if you have any underlying conditions. Discuss adapting the steps of the Self-Health Program with your doctor, if indicated by your condition.

❑ Take the Self-Health Evaluations, and record your health history. Review your familial and personal health histories.

❑ Set a firm date to start the program. Once you establish the date, don't let any excuses postpone your progress.

CHAPTER 6

The Momentum Month: Month One of the Holistic Self-Health Program

The first month is the time to establish your commitment to the program. You need to begin gently and slowly, but with strong and steady resolve. Consistency and determination are keys to building self-health and achieving the goals of the program. Keep your eyes on the prize: a renewed sense of energy, purpose, and well-being that awaits you.

During each biweekly period you'll be starting new activities but also continuing with those you've already initiated. Once these healthful patterns are incorporated into your life, it's important to continue them for the duration of the program (and, we hope, much longer). First you put down the foundation; then you build on your progress.

When you're ready to start the program, read through this chapter once for an overall picture of the first month. Then review the steps, and plan how you will accomplish them.

Congratulations on starting your new life!

WEEKS ONE AND TWO

Evaluate Your Triangle and Decide Where to Focus

All of us need to nourish all three sides of our Holistic Triangles constantly in order to achieve balance and total well-being. But during the program we should also be aware of what needs extra attention.

During the first few days set aside some time to look at the results of your Self-Health Evaluations. This will give you an indication of which sides are strong and which need more work.

You can also evaluate your Triangle by reviewing the health problems you've had in the past and any messages your body is giving you now. All the sides are connected and affect the way we feel, but certain maladies indicate weaknesses on certain sides of the Triangle:

- Weakness on the physical side may be indicated by frequent injuries, aches and pains, bodily tension, low energy level, and feeling out of shape.
- Diseases, gastrointestinal distress, fluctuating levels of energy, and headaches are signals of weakness on the chemical side.
- Anxiety, confusion, poor concentration, lack of faith, low self-esteem, and depression indicate lack of nourishment on the mental/spiritual side but often also have a strong chemical component.

If the majority of your problems are on one or another of these sides, this signals where to give extra nourishment. Restoring optimum nourishment will help your body heal itself.

You can also contemplate which sides of your Triangle are already powerful and receiving plenty of nourishment. If you're very strong on one side, focus attention on nourishing the less developed areas of your Triangle.

This doesn't mean you'll neglect a side if it is already strong; it means the program will take you even further. If you're in good shape now, you can get closer to your physical peak. If you're a healthy eater, you can go on an extended juice fast (see page 188). Whatever side is strong can be taken to a higher level, and whatever side is undernourished can be given special attention.

The tendency is to do more work on the side that is already powerful and to resist confronting the weak areas. You'll need to make a plan to avoid this common pitfall, and remember: Where there is resistance there is tremendous potential.

At this point you should establish a Self-Health Notebook to chart your progress during the program. You can put your Self-Health Evaluation questionnaires inside this notebook, and use it to plan and record your Self-Health activities.

List "Mental/Spiritual Side," "Chemical Side," and "Physical Side" on each page. Referring to the results of your Self-Health Evaluations, and your own thoughts, write an assessment of each side of your Triangle. Include a determination assessment of which sides you think are stronger and weaker and need special care. This written evaluation allows you to be your own doctor, recording your condition on your own health chart.

Create a Weekly Nourishment Plan

A Weekly Nourishment Plan is a written plan on which you list all the ways you will nourish each side of your Triangle that week. Here is an example of a plan:

Weekly Nourishment Plan

Mental/spiritual side:
Do Bathing Ritual, including Healing Moment, every day.
Practice deep breathing in spare moments.
Go to bookstore, and buy books on visualization and massage.
Try healing visualization for that annoying lower back pain.

Chemical side:
Have soy milk and whole grain cereal instead of my usual breakfast.

Bring a banana or plum to work for morning munchies.

Make chili with beans instead of meat for dinner.

Cut out the afternoon cup of coffee. Later in week, put half the usual amount in filter for morning cup.

Get the cookies out of the house so I won't be tempted.

Keep up my Daily Diet Report (see page 134).

Physical side:

Try to stop crossing my legs.

Stretch when I get home from work.

Go for a brisk twenty-minute walk at least three times a week.

Look into joining the Y for swimming.

At the end of the week review your Weekly Nourishment Plan, and check off how many of your planned activities you accomplished. Then create a plan for the following week.

It's also helpful to record your activities on the Physical and and Mental/Spiritual Nourishment forms on page 133. You can make copies of these forms, three-hole-punch the pages, and include them in your Self-Health Notebook. This offers a quick and efficient way to chart your progress.

These written exercises are very helpful for most people; they provide a structure that makes the Self-Health Program more manageable. However, if you hate making lists or keeping records, don't let this aspect of the program stop you from progressing. You can plan your activities and keep a list in your head, if necessary. Don't let technicalities slow you down; be creative and adapt the program to suit your personality.

Luxuriate in the Bathing Ritual

The Bathing Ritual is the ideal preparation for the other activities of the program. Try to do it as many days of the week as you can.

Please review the Bathing Ritual instructions on page 219.

While you are in the bath, picture the current state of your Holistic Triangle, and visualize exactly what you'll do to nurture each side today. Ask yourself these questions:

Am I going to let my environment and work control me, or am I going to control my environment and take steps to nourish myself?

How am I going to nourish the mental/spiritual side of my Triangle today? The chemical side? The physical side?

What obstacles and difficulties might I encounter when working on my program? How will I overcome them and continue to make progress?

Nourish Your Mental/Spiritual Side

To build your commitment to the program and your faith in the innate healing force, you need to have a thorough knowledge of the truth about health. Continue to educate yourself and nourish your mental side throughout the three months of the program.

The books you choose may be about spiritual topics, religion, affirmations and visualizations, self-healing, yoga, meditation, relaxation, nutrition, vegetarianism, vitamins, herbology, raw juicing, fasting, the history of health care, alternative health care modalities, massage, exercise, or any other topic that builds your mental/spiritual side. Suggestions are on pages 229–232.

It's also vital to nurture your spirituality during the program. Take some time to review the methods of developing faith and nourishing your spiritual side in Chapter 2. Then decide which practices you will include in your program. Try to spend some time on your spiritual self, at least a few Healing Moments, every day during the program.

Practice Positive Thinking

The number one goal during the first month of the program is to build your foundation of self-love, self-esteem, and faith in your innate healing force. Throughout the month, try continually to affirm in your thoughts and actions that you deserve unconditional love. Promise to show your self-love by nourishing your Triangle and staying with the Self-Health Program.

You can use affirmations and visualizations to confirm your commitment to the program, enhance your self-esteem and self-love, and work toward healing specific problems. These techniques can help positive thinking become a natural reflex. See details on page 44.

Start Your Daily Diet Report

The purpose of the Daily Diet Report is to give you a clear picture of your toxic input and your healthy input. Even if you choose not to do the other written exercises, try to do this report. If you resist writing down the truth about what you consume, it probably means there's something you don't want to see.

The Daily Diet Report should include everything you eat and drink and the number of servings. Use the form on page 134 or create your own. Fill in the report at the end of each day or the following morning. Don't let it go longer than the next morning, or you may forget what you had.

At the end of the week make a list of all the toxins you consumed, referring to the list of the Top Ten Toxins in Chapter 3. It will give you guidance when you start to reduce your intake of toxins.

Increase Healthy Intake

It's vital that you consume plenty of healthy food and drink to supply fuel for the activities of the Self-Health Program and reduce the craving for toxins. During the first month increase your consumption of raw fruits and vegetables, whole grains, and nonmeat protein, such as legumes, nuts, and seeds. Reviewing the suggestions in Chapter 3 can give you some ideas on wholesome nourishment. Vegetarian cookbooks are also full of ideas.

Try to follow the pattern of eating six small meals a day rather than three large ones. Lunch should be the largest meal, while dinner is light.

Start a new habit of keeping a glass of pure water at your side throughout the day. Try to drink at least six glasses a day of water during the first month of the program. You may find it helpful to carry a plastic pint or quart bottle of water with you.

It's also recommended you take high-quality multivitamin/mineral supplements made from natural food sources throughout the program. These will address any deficiencies you may have and fortify your chemical side.

Do Aerobic Exercise Three Times a Week

Start your aerobic exercise program gently with an activity you know you can do and you think you'll enjoy. Don't be intimidated by the term "aerobics," which can bring to mind impossibly fit people jumping up and down for an hour. Remember, walking and swimming are also highly beneficial aerobic activities.

Even if you've been neglecting your physical side for years, you can make a determination to walk three times a week. If walking is not enough of a challenge, choose a more dynamic aerobic activity. Refer to the Aerobic Choices for Fitness Levels 1–4 on pages 75–76 for guidance.

Chapter 4 can also give you an idea of the pros and cons of different exercises. You may want to try a variety of forms and then stick with what you like best, or you may choose to do several different aerobic workouts each week. You can swim one day, walk one day, and dance one day—whatever gets you going and keeps you moving.

Exercise researchers have found twenty minutes to be the minimal amount of time to gain the full benefits of aerobic activity. If your physical side is weak, you may need to work up to this time by doing ten minutes twice a day, with rest periods in between, for the first week or two. Then try to do fifteen minutes straight the next week. The goal by the end of the first month of the program is twenty minutes of aerobic exercise at least three times a week.

Before starting any aerobic exercise, review the danger signs on page 76. If you experience any of these problems, consult your health professional. Whenever you work out, be highly aware of your breathing. If you become out of breath or have difficulty speaking while you are exercising, slow down. A comfortable respiratory rate should be maintained, with your inhalations and exhalations in sync with the exercise. Monitor your pulse according to the formula on page 210.

Keep in mind that the law of inertia may make it difficult to get started, but once you get moving, aerobic exercise is *fun.* Your endorphins will be stimulated, and you'll feel a natural "high." You'll gain confidence, feel more energetic, and have a stronger heart as a result of your workouts.

Begin Musculoskeletal Exercises

Another goal on the physical side is to begin the practice of muscular development exercises three times each week, alternating with aerobic exercise. If you have been neglecting your physical side, the musculoskeletal workout can be gentle and modified. Consistency is the primary concern; in later months of the program you can build up duration and intensity.

The musculoskeletal exercise sequence on page 211 provides a basic workout. Depending on your condition, you may need to start with only the leg raises the first week, add the sit-up sequence the second week, and then include the push-ups and jumping jacks.

For every action there is a reaction, and once you start exercising, weaknesses and problems you did not realize were present may surface. Pay attention to the messages your body sends you. Don't give up, but modify your exercise program until you've built up your physical side. Consult with a professional if you experience anything worse than minor body aches.

Challenge your body, but respect it. Don't push too hard or you may have a backlash in the form of injury or giving up on the program. You need to find your own delicate balance between being lazy and pressing yourself too hard.

You can keep a detailed record of your exercise activities on the Physical Nourishment form. This will help you see how your endurance builds during the program and will give you positive reinforcement.

Include Stretching and Deep Breathing in Your Daily Routine

The stretching exercises in the bathtub will get you started on your flexibility program, but you should also do stretches before and after your aerobic and musculoskeletal sessions. If you limber up conscientiously, you'll be less vulnerable to injury and pain.

It's suggested you do a complete stretching session, as outlined on page 215, or practice yoga once or twice a week. You may want to do this on your own or join a class.

The stretching session is an excellent time to practice deep breathing and increase your oxygen intake. You can also practice deep breathing while you're driving, waiting, or taking a "breather" at work. Stretching is one of the perks of the Self-Health Program, and you should enjoy it whenever possible.

Rest and Relaxation

One of the ways to show self-love is to give yourself enough time to sleep. Throughout the program you'll probably need seven to eight hours of solid sleep each night. Try not to oversleep, for this can make you lethargic and interfere with your progress.

Since so much of your life is spent sleeping, it pays to invest in a good, quality firm mattress to give your body the support it needs. If you're a stomach sleeper, begin training yourself to sleep on your side or your back to reduce strain on your lower back, spine, and neck. If you sleep with two pillows, try sleeping with one to reduce stress on your cervical vertebrae.

Since you'll be challenging the physical side of your body during the program, it's beneficial to practice Total Body Relaxation at least twice a week. This will enhance your body awareness and reduce aches and pains from exercise.

One day a week can be your vacation from all exercise except stretching. On this day of rest you might treat yourself to extra physical nourishment, such as a sauna or Jacuzzi, a self-massage or a professional massage, or a longer session in the bathtub.

THE THIRD AND FOURTH WEEKS

Reminder: During these weeks, in addition to the new activities detailed below, continue with all the healthy actions of the first two weeks:

- Weekly Nourishment Plans
- Mental/spiritual nourishment through reading and spiritual practices
- Bathing Ritual
- Daily Diet Reports
- Increase in natural food and water intake
- Aerobic exercise, musculoskeletal exercise, and stretching on a regular basis
- Rest and relaxation

Keep the momentum going!

Reduce Toxic Intake

The third week of the program is the time to start reducing the amount of toxins you consume. Refer to your list of toxins from your Daily Diet Report. Write down in your Weekly Nourishment Plan what toxins you plan to reduce or eliminate each day.

You are not expected to eliminate completely all toxins during the first month of the program; the major focus is on building up your mental/spiritual side so you have the commitment and knowledge to detoxify in the second month. But you should aim to *reduce* toxic input during the first month. The degree of reduction will depend on the current state of your chemical side. A reduction of 50 percent is a general goal, but if you find yourself doing better, more power to your Triangle!

When you begin reducing your intake of "everyday" toxins, such as sugar, white bread, dairy products, or meat, expect to encounter a lot of resistance within yourself. It helps to read more about these particular toxins so as to reinforce the reasons why you need to eliminate them. Also keep in mind that your tastes will evolve, and by the end of the second month you'll find your-self less attracted to toxins you now crave. You can educate the chemical side of your Triangle as well as the mental side.

Seek Support to Overcome Addictions, If Necessary

If you are addicted to nicotine, alcohol, or drugs, it's crucial to seek out support for the withdrawal process.

If you have a drug or alcohol addiction, you can find out about local meetings of Alcoholics Anonymous and other twelve-step groups, or look into professional treatment programs. A trusted holistic health care professional can also be a resource for the re-habilitation process. If you have a nicotine addiction, consider joining one of the quit-smoking groups that are run by many state lung associations. Look into hypnotherapy or acupuncture for ad-ditional support.

Learn what meetings, programs, and professional help are available in your area, and the schedules, locations, and costs. Try to visit the group or meet with the health practitioner to de-termine if this is the right source of support for you.

By the end of the first month of the program set a firm date to go to the meeting, enter the program, or consult the health pro-fessional within the next ten days. Make a vow to do whatever is necessary to overcome your addiction, and strengthen your re-solve with prayer, Healing Moments, and affirmations.

Become Aware of Your Posture

During the first month set aside time to become aware of your posture when sitting and standing. Study yourself in a mirror, or have a friend take a few front and side photographs to get a clear view of your standing posture. See if your neck is craning for-ward, if you are slumping, if you are hyperextended or swaying to one side. Then you can make a mental note to work on pulling up and aligning yourself.

When sitting, notice if you habitually cross your legs. If you do, you may need to put up written reminders near your chairs for the first month to undo the leg-crossing habit.

See if your chairs allow you to keep your feet flat on the floor and your knees level to or slightly higher than your hips. Are you sitting up tall or rounding your lower back? Determine if you need to get an ergonomically designed chair for your workplace or better chairs for home.

Good posture takes muscular strength as well as awareness, and it may be some time before you can maintain it throughout the day. But during the first month you can start being conscious of your posture and making the effort to improve it. Soon you'll have more strength to maintain good posture, and doing so will give you more energy and power.

CHECKLIST FOR THE MOMENTUM MONTH

❑ Evaluate your Holistic Triangle and start your Self-Health Notebook.

❑ Write out your Daily Nourishment Plan each week.

❑ Start your day the holistic way with the Bathing Ritual.

❑ Nourish your mental/spiritual side with reading, spiritual practices, affirmations, and visualizations.

❑ Keep a Daily Diet Report, and list all toxins.

❑ Eat more fruits, vegetables, grains, and nonmeat protein. Drink at least six glasses of water a day.

❑ Take high-quality multivitamin/mineral supplements.

❑ Sleep seven to eight hours a day.

❑ Do the Total Body Relaxation and breathing exercises frequently.

❑ Stretch every day.

❑ Do aerobic exercise three times a week, gradually building up duration and intensity.

❑ Do musculoskeletal exercise three times a week, gradually building up repetitions.

❑ Start to reduce your intake of toxins.

❑ Plan to join a support group or seek professional help to overcome addictions, if necessary.

❑ Become aware of your posture and work to improve it.

❑ Think about how much you've done at the end of the month, and give yourself a heartfelt pat on the back!

Physical Nourishment Report

Physical Side

Date: From _____ To_____

	1st Day	2nd Day	3rd Day	4th Day	5th Day	6th Day	7th Day
Cardiovascular (Aerobic)							
Time							
Musculoskeletal							
Time							
Stretching/ Limbering							
Time							
Rest (Sleep)							
Time							

Mental/Spiritual Nourishment

Mental/Spiritual Foundation Side

Approximate time per seven days

Daily Diet Report

Chemical Side

Date: From _____ To _____

Meals	1st Day	2nd Day	3rd Day	4th Day	5th Day	6th Day	7th Day
Breakfast							
Time							
Snack							
Time							
Lunch							
Time							
Snack							
Time							
Dinner							
Time							
Snack							
Time							

CHAPTER 7

The Cleansing Month: Month Two of the Holistic Self-Health Program

The primary goal of the second month is to detoxify your entire system by eliminating toxins and through raw-juice fasting. You'll also continue to build your physical side with a balanced exercise program and get plenty of mental/spiritual nourishment.

This is a cleansing month, when you'll get rid of chemical toxins *and* negative thoughts and habits. If you are overweight, it's likely that you'll lose fat and gain muscle. You'll emerge feeling leaner and cleaner, both mentally and physically.

The second month of the program requires sharp focus and organization. Your Weekly Nourishment Plan should include a specific timetable for giving up each toxin. Even if you decided not to write the plan during the first month, it's recommended you write down a timetable for giving up each toxin. Otherwise you may fall into the "I'll start tomorrow" trap. Put your detoxification schedule in writing, and sign it, as a contract with yourself.

For some people with some toxins, it's easier to go cold turkey, while for others, a gradual withdrawal is more feasible. You don't want to make it too gradual, however. *Aim to eliminate all toxins by the end of the second week of this month.*

If you don't succeed with this schedule, you can still continue with the program and make progress. But if you set your mind on this goal, you may surprise yourself with your success. You can do it!

You also need to plan ahead for two major events during this month: a one-day juice fast, preferably at the beginning of the third week, and a three-day juice fast at the end of the month. Try to schedule these fasts on weekends or at times when you won't be under particular stress at work. Circle your fast dates in red on your calendar, and promise yourself you'll stick to your plan.

If you do not already own a raw juicer, you'll need to purchase one for the Cleansing Month. This is an essential health appliance that will allow you to enjoy the benefits of raw juices throughout the month as well as during fast days.

WEEKS FIVE AND SIX

During the first month it was recommended you seek appropriate support if you needed to overcome an addiction to alcohol, drugs, or nicotine. The first week of the second month is the time to start going to meetings, support groups, treatment programs, or the health practitioner who will help you through withdrawal.

Even if the toxins you need to eliminate are socially sanctioned substances, such as caffeine, sugar, dairy products, or meat, it's helpful to have support. If possible, enlist the assistance of your spouse or a trusted friend or relative. Be sure to pick a person who believes in detoxification and understands the dangers of the Top Ten Toxins. If there's no one in your personal life who understands, you can ask your holistic health care provider to be your support person.

Often it's easier to lie to ourselves than to people we respect. Having someone who cares check on the progress of your program can be a motivation for good behavior. Tell your support person exactly what toxin you plan to eliminate and when. Ask her or him to inquire how you're doing with your plan every few days and to encourage you to stick with the detoxification program. Ultimately it's up to you, but a caring support person can help you stay the course when the going gets rough.

Review Healthy Alternatives to the Top Ten Toxins

As you eliminate toxins, you can replace many of them with nourishing substitutes. After a transition period, you'll probably find these replacements much more appetizing than the toxins. Here is a refresher on Healthy Alternatives.

1. Toxin: Sugar and Sugar Products
   Alternatives
   Small amounts of raw, unfiltered honey, maple syrup, barley malt syrup, rice syrup, and diluted fruit juice
   Six small meals a day, with a variety of wholesome foods, to maintain blood sugar level and reduce craving

Note: During sugar withdrawal, limit consumption of fruit juices, and avoid white flour products and white potatoes.

2. Toxin: White Flour and Refined Carbohydrates
   Alternatives
   Foods made with whole wheat flour, buckwheat flour, rice flour, rye flour, and cornmeal
   Pastas, breads, and cereals made from whole grains (be sure they do not contain sugar)
   Brown rice and wild rice
   Couscous, millet, bulgur wheat, buckwheat, quinoa, amaranth, and other whole grains

3. Toxin: Dairy Products
   Alternatives
   Soy beverage, almond beverage, and rice beverage

Almond butter, filbert butter, cashew butter, pecan butter, and apple butter

Cheeses, yogurt, and mayonnaise made from soy

For calcium: greens, beans, and seeds

4. Toxin: Meat

Alternatives

Legumes (beans, peas and lentils)

Tofu and other soybean products

Nuts in moderation

High- to medium-protein plant foods

Limited amounts of fish, organic poultry, and eggs (no more than one serving per day)

5. Toxin: Food Additives (Including Salt)

Alternatives

Fresh food with its natural flavor

Prepared food bought only in health food stores with labels checked carefully to see there are no additives

Foods seasoned with a variety of herb and spices instead of added salt

6. Toxin: Caffeine

Alternatives

Small, frequent, nourishing meals to keep up energy levels

Oxygen boosters—exercise and deep breathing—to increase energy

Fruit juices (diluted), herbal teas, and beverages made from roasted grains and seeds

7. Toxin: Nicotine

Alternatives

Quitting smoking with support of groups, clinics, acupuncture, and raw-juice fasting

Increased oxygen intake with deep breathing and exercise

8. Toxin: Alcohol

Alternatives

Sobriety with support of Alcoholics Anonymous, treatment programs, and holistic health care

Development of spirituality; practice of meditation and relaxation techniques

Wholesome foods and increased vitamin/mineral supplementation for nutritional support

Diluted fruit juices with carbonated water, fruit punches, and sparkling cider

9. Toxin: Drugs

Alternatives

Maintenance of health by nourishing Holistic Triangle

Meditation and spiritual practices

Exercise for release of endorphins

Prevention of need for prescription drugs through proper diet, exercise, and positive thinking

Natural health care, such as chiropractic, nutritional counseling, acupuncture, and massage

Limited use of healing herbs and homeopathic remedies

10. Toxin: Environmental Toxins

Alternatives

Organic fruits and vegetables

Natural, chemical-free personal products

Chemical-free cleaning products

Checking for toxins in home, such as radon and lead paint, with removal if necessary

Assessment of health hazards in workplace, and steps taken to correct problems

Review the list of toxins you made during the first month of the program. Be sure to add any you missed, such as environmental poisons, prescription drugs, cigarettes, and other nonfood toxins. This is your hit list: the enemies standing between you and well-being. It may sound melodramatic to call a piece of apple pie or a beer an "enemy." But during the program you need to view even sociably acceptable toxins as enemies of your health.

After the program, if you choose to indulge in toxins occasionally, that's up to you. It won't do you any good, but it probably won't do you much harm. But for these three months you're committed to completely detoxifying and filling yourself with love and healthy input. *If you want to maximize results and awake your full healing force, you need to give your body a complete cleansing.*

Take a blank page in your Self-Health Notebook and draw a line down the center. On one side write "Toxin," and on the other side, "Healthy Alternatives." Write down all your toxins on one side of the page and the healthier options on the opposite side. In addition to the choices listed here, be inventive and write down your own ideas.

As you give up each toxin, cross it off in your notebook. The other side of the page will remind you to reward yourself with healthy nourishment.

HALT Your Toxic Habits

In addiction therapy there is an acronym: HALT. Four triggers for substance abuse are: **H**unger **A**nger **L**oneliness **T**iredness. These triggers represent lack of nourishment on the different sides of the Triangle: hunger—chemical side; anger and loneliness—mental/spiritual side; tiredness—physical side. Boredom and tension are two other triggers of which you should be aware.

When you have the desire to indulge in a toxin, reflect on whether you are experiencing one of these feelings. Then, before you reflexively give in to the urge, think of how you can overcome your discomfort in a healthy, loving way. Here are some ideas:

Hunger

Eat small portions of healthy foods six times a day. Concentrate on your meals while you are eating. Chew slowly and thoroughly to make the food last. Drink eight glasses of water between meals.

Anger

Anger usually comes from fear. Work on your mental/spiritual foundation to reduce fear and learn to be more forgiving. Remember we're all imperfect, yet we're all deserving of unconditional love. For immediate alleviation of fear and anger, try deep breathing. Above all, don't consume a toxin that will make you angry at yourself. Do something truly nourishing that will help you be strong enough to rise above anger.

Loneliness

The more you love yourself, the greater opportunity you have to attract loving people into your life. However, loneliness is a complex problem with societal as well as personal factors, and there may be times when you lack fulfilling companionship. Try to develop healthy coping mechanisms for loneliness instead of seeking comfort in toxins. For example, join a spiritual or religious group where you may find kindred spirits, go to an exercise class where you may make friends, or do volunteer work with people who need your help.

Tiredness

People often turn to toxins to give them temporary lifts and then are left lower than before when their blood sugar levels crash. A diet of six nutritious minimeals a day can lift you out of this cycle and help you avoid using toxins to overcome fatigue. Deep breathing, yoga, and exercise can also boost your energy level naturally.

Boredom

During the program it's unlikely you'll have time to be bored since you'll be busy with activities that stimulate your mind and body. These nourishing activities can become lifelong habits to keep you from becoming bored and turning to toxins to fill your leisure hours.

If you often get bored at your job, try to become more engaged in your work and create new challenges. If your job does not have any room for growth, change, or intellectual stimulation, you may need a career change. The month after you finish the program, when you'll be in peak mental and physical condition, may be a smart time to make a move.

Tension

Keep in mind that the very toxin you are reaching for to relieve tension may have a rebound effect and actually increase anxiety. Try to react with a healthy coping mechanism instead of a toxic crutch.

The more you love yourself and nourish your mental/spiritual side, the less power tension and anxiety will have over your life. However, you also need balanced nourishment on the physical side to relieve tension. Exercise is a potent tension reliever, and deep breathing is also effective.

Whenever you reach for a toxin, HALT! Reflect on whether you are hungry, angry, lonely, tired, bored, or tense. Think of a way you can alleviate your condition in a healthy, self-loving way. Then do it. Gradually, healthy actions will become habitual, and you won't need toxins as coping mechanisms.

Drink Raw Juices Throughout the Month

If you do not already own a juicer, purchase one at the beginning of the second month of the program. Later in the month you'll be accelerating your detoxification with raw-juice fasts. But throughout the month you should drink three glasses of raw juice each day: two vegetable juices and one fruit juice. The enzymes in the raw juices will fortify your entire Holistic Triangle and give you the energy to detoxify.

During this month of detoxification it's highly recommended that you buy organic produce and avoid the pesticides and herbicides in most supermarket produce.

Fruit juices should always be distilled with 50 percent water. If you are withdrawing from a heavy sugar habit, avoid the juices of the sweeter fruits and have no more than six ounces of fruit juice each day, in the morning. Also, be aware that citrus juices can cause skin problems and acne for allergic people. If you have a history of citrus allergies or find yourself with skin symptoms after drinking citrus juices, select other produce.

Green juices made from spinach, kale, parsley, alfalfa, and other green vegetables contain chlorophyll, which is effective in the cleansing process. One of the most potent green drinks is wheatgrass juice, which requires special equipment to produce. Your home juicer may not work to supply this, but you can buy wheatgrass juice fresh in some health food stores or in frozen or powdered form. One ounce of this strong detoxifier is enough to produce an effect.

Raw juices made from vegetables help remove wastes from the body and supply precious antioxidants, amino acids, vitamins, and minerals. Sprouts are highly nutritious and can be added to any of your vegetable drinks.

It's best to drink your raw juices immediately, but if you want to bring them to work, you can store them in an airtight container in a refrigerator or a thermos for up to twelve hours. If necessary, you can prepare them on weekends and store in the freezer.

You can try some of the raw-juice suggestions in Chapter 3 and experiment with your own combinations. We recommend highly that you drink at least one of the detoxification recipes on page 191 each day. These special combinations are designed to nourish and cleanse the lungs, liver, skin, immune system, and vascular system.

Support Cleansing with Energy Foods, Water, and Supplements

During withdrawal from such toxins as sugar and caffeine, it's crucial to maintain a steady stream of nutrients to reduce cravings. Eating six small meals spaced throughout the day will help keep your blood sugar and energy levels steady. Raw-juice drinks can constitute two of these meals, especially if you want to lose weight. Be sure to include a hearty green salad on a daily basis and a whole grain dish every day.

Be adventurous during this month. Try new grains and fruits and vegetables. Eat for the health of it, not just the taste of it.

Imagine your body being nourished on a deeper level; focus on the energy and sustenance from the food.

Drink at least six glasses of filtered water throughout the day to promote cleansing and reduce the tendency to overeat.

Supplements can also support withdrawal from toxins and detoxification. Your holistic health care provider can give you specific guidance on vitamins, minerals, herbs, and amino acids that benefit your particular condition. You can also refer to page 208 for guidelines on supplements and herbs for detoxification.

Eliminate or Reduce Medications

This is the month to stop leaning on quick fixes and commit yourself to the hard work of looking for long-term solutions to health problems without drugs.

Holistic health books organized according to ailment can teach you about alternatives to medications. It's worthwhile including such books in your home library and learning how to utilize natural remedies and prevention. You can refer to page 207 for natural alternatives to several common nonprescription drugs.

The Cleansing Month is the time to eliminate or reduce dependency on prescription drugs as well as over-the-counter items. Schedule a consultation with your doctor to discuss the possibility of reducing or eliminating medications if you take them regularly. Whether or not you can do this will depend on the severity and chronicity of your condition and how long you have been on the medication. But the majority of people can eventually improve their health to a point where drugs are no longer required.

It may take much longer than three months of the program to strengthen your Holistic Triangle sufficiently so that medication is no longer needed, and in rare cases it may never be possible. But it is your right to have your health care practitioner explain the reasons for your medication and carefully consider if you can reduce or discontinue it.

In many cases medication is freely dispensed because it seems an easier solution than major lifestyle changes. Since nearly all drugs have side effects, it's critical to examine every possible natural alternative instead of blindly continuing to swallow your medicine.

Be Prepared for a Healing Crisis

As you withdraw from toxins and your body begins to cleanse itself, you may undergo a healing crisis. Common symptoms include headaches, coughing and clogged sinuses, skin eruptions, gastrointestinal distress, diarrhea, fatigue, irritability, and depression. These messages show the powerful physiological power the toxin is exerting on your mind/body. The more extreme the healing crisis, the more necessary the detoxification.

Symptoms during a healing crisis need to be monitored by your health care professional. But they are not a signal that you should stop the program and turn back to your old habits. Call on your mental/spiritual stamina to keep going. Let the symptoms serve as motivation and a reminder of how much you need to detoxify.

Keep in mind that with most addictions the first three days are the worst, and after this period the physical symptoms usually subside. Take one day at a time, and give yourself plenty of support on all three sides of your Holistic Triangle.

When you give up caffeine, even if your habit is as little as one or two cups of coffee a day, you may experience a withdrawal headache, fatigue, and irritability. These symptoms indicate the serious nature of the ubiquitous caffeine addiction. Don't take aspirin or any other type of pain reliever to relieve your discomfort; this will only prolong your dependency. Instead you can turn to holistic treatments:

- Massage of acupressure points
- Alternating hot and cold compresses (see page 228)
- Exercise, particularly swimming
- Chiropractic care
- Acupuncture

Acupuncture is also recommended if you are overcoming an addiction to drugs, alcohol, or nicotine. It is often effective in easing withdrawal symptoms and is utilized in some progressive rehabilitation programs.

Chiropractic adjustments to maximize the flow of energy through your nerves is another therapeutic alternative during withdrawal. Professional Swedish massage, lymphatic massage, and reflexology can help move waste material through the system and facilitate lymphatic drainage.

Plenty of sleep is required during the detoxification process. Your liver and other organs are working hard to eliminate years of accumulated debris, and you may need extra hours of sleep or quiet, restful time by yourself.

Be sure you have a supply of fresh air when you are indoors: an open window, not just an air conditioner. And try to get outside for short walks whenever possible. You may need to slow down your exercise program during a health crisis, but continue to stretch and do some movement.

Drink eight glasses of filtered water during a detoxification process to help flush through the toxins. Eat steadily but lightly, mostly raw fruits and vegetables.

If You Relapse, Try Again

Toxins have a powerful effect on our mental/spiritual base and often sabotage our decisions and resolve. It's very common to be unable to give up a toxin during the first attempt or to give it up for a short time and then relapse.

If you fail to eliminate the toxin or have a relapse, don't let this throw you off the Self-Health Program.

Be a loving, understanding friend to yourself. Forgive yourself, and reaffirm your unconditional self-love. Don't let a setback make you feel like a complete failure; review the progress you've made in the program and the steps you've accomplished. Focus on your successes as a reminder that you *can* change.

Next, consider why you couldn't give up the toxin or started taking it again. What stood in your way? Was it a physical craving? A psychological need? An escape? Plan how you can keep these pitfalls from sabotaging your progress. What extra nourishment on every side of your Triangle can give you the strength to free yourself of the toxin?

Plan extra nourishment and support during your next attempt to give up the toxin. Call on the powerful healing force of love and the Creator to give you support. Reaffirm your commitment to the program and your faith in your innate healing power. Set a firm date and try again.

Nourish Your Physical Side

The Holistic Self-Health Program is a progressive plan; each month you add to the previous month's accomplishments. During the second month you should continue to nurture your physical side with these activities:

- Bathing Ritual and bathtub exercises nearly every day
- Additional stretching before and after musculoskeletal and aerobic sessions
- Musculoskeletal exercise three times a week
- Aerobic exercise at least three times a week, for at least twenty minutes each session

If you want to do more exercise than this schedule indicates, go for it. Vary your exercise program if you're starting to get bored. Increase the intensity of your aerobic exercise if you feel ready. Add weight training to your musculoskeletal workout if you want to build up.

Listen to your body, and don't overdo it. "No pain no gain" is a fallacy. A pain-free, fun, and natural exercise program is more likely to become a permanent part of your life. By this second month of exercising, you should be seeing and feeling the benefits, and these will inspire you to keep moving.

WEEKS SEVEN AND EIGHT

During the last two weeks of the Cleansing Month continue to nourish your mental/spiritual side with stimulating reading material, spiritual practices, and positive thinking. You should also carry on with your aerobic and musculoskeletal exercises, with the exception of the fast days, when you can reduce activity. The highlight of this period will be the three-day raw-juice fast, which will shift your inner healing force into high gear.

Go on a One-Day Raw-Juice Fast

The best time to schedule your one-day fast is at the beginning of the third week of the second month. By this date you should have reduced or eliminated most of your toxins. Even if you have not, however, it's likely you can still go on a one-day juice fast, provided you consult your holistic doctor first. The fast may well be the day you finally learn you can live without toxins.

Remember, *raw-juice fasting is not starvation*. In fact, drinking raw juices throughout the day can provide more nourishment than the Standard American Diet.

Juice fasting is a powerful healing tool that will help you cleanse your body of years of toxic buildup and also benefit your mental/spiritual side. On your first fast day you'll gain confidence and learn you don't have to be a slave to your habits. You'll also learn to disassociate a certain degree of hunger from punishment and realize that cutting back on food is actually a *reward* for your body.

Try to schedule the fast for a day when you'll be home so you'll have easy access to your juicer. The day before your fast, eat only raw fruits and vegetables, and drink several fresh juices and the Fiber Broth to start the cleansing process.

A one-day juice fast lasts for twenty-four hours—from the first morning when you wake up to the second morning. It is not effective to fast all day and then eat dinner; you need to give your body a rest for a full day and night.

On the day of the fast drink six to ten ounces of a freshly made raw juice every two hours, until a few hours before bedtime. This should be seven glasses of juice: four or five primarily vegetable juices and two or three fruit juices. Start with a fruit juice for your first drink of the morning. Include at least three of the special detoxification recipes in your juice menu.

While raw-juice fasting, you won't need to drink as much water as usual, but still drink one or two glasses a day. It is not necessary to take your vitamin and mineral supplements while you are juice fasting, since you'll be getting high concentrations of nutrients in the juices. Don't chew gum or anything else while fasting.

Start with the Bathing Ritual and bathtub exercises in the morning. Stretching, yoga, walking, or other light exercise are fine while juice fasting, but strenuous aerobics and musculoskeletal workouts are not recommended. Healing Moments, relaxation practices, meditation, and communion with nature are ideal activities.

You may want to keep a diary of your one-day fast in your Self-Help Notebook. Record how you feel, what cravings you experience, the good and bad moments. This will help you identify possible stumbling blocks for the grand finale of your detoxification month: the three-day juice fast.

Go on a Three-Day Juice Fast

Your three-day juice fast should be scheduled at the end of the second month of the program. By this point you've eliminated most toxins from your diet. You've had a month of sun foods, raw juices, and supplements. You've learned you can gain control of your appetite by completing the one-day juice fast. You're ready to activate your inner healing potential with the three-day juice fast.

Before embarking on this fast, check again with your doctor to be sure you have no conditions that preclude juice fasting. If you have a history of diabetes, kidney disease, or another major illness or are on medication, you need to consult with your doctor and find out if fasting is safe and what special precautions you may need to take. Even if you are in the best of health, have a holistic health professional on call in case you experience any unusual symptoms during the fast.

Have a serving of the Fiber Broth each day between your one-day and three-day juice fast. For two days before the second fast, eat only raw fruits, vegetables, nuts, and seeds; drink plenty of water; and take supplements. Once you are on the juice fast, you don't need supplements and can drink less water than usual.

Each day of the fast drink a raw juice every two hours, starting with a fruit juice in the morning. Include at least three of the detoxification juice recipes each day. Add a teaspoon of spirulina powder to two or three of your juice drinks daily.

Each day of the fast, drink one or two cups of healing teas, such as pau d'arco and echinacea, and at least one glass of distilled water.

It's important to have a bowel movement during each day of the juice fast to continue the inner cleansing process. But since the peristaltic response will not be stimulated by any food, you'll probably need an enema on the second morning.

Use distilled lukewarm water in the enema bag, with a little lemon juice added (unless you have a citrus allergy). Insert the tube with your head down and bottom up. After the fluid insertion, lie on your right side and gently massage the right side of your abdomen. Turn on your back, and massage the center of your abdomen; then turn to the left, and massage the left side.

Be sure to place a small stool or a couple of telephone books under your feet when you are on the toilet bowl to simulate the squatting position. If there is any blood or excess mucus in your feces, notify your health care provider. These signs do not necessarily mean your fast needs to be discontinued, but you may require special therapeutic juices.

After the enema you can relax in the bath, perhaps adding some soothing oils.

On fast days you need to brush your tongue as thoroughly as your teeth. Buildup of white mucus on your tongue while fasting is to be expected; it's a sign your body is cleaning itself out. Brush your tongue with a natural toothpaste; then wipe it from the back to the front with a terry-cloth washcloth until it's clean.

Fasting is used as a spiritual tradition in many cultures, and juice fast days are an excellent time to give extra attention to your mental/spiritual side. Meditation, relaxation, affirmations, visualization, Healing Moments, and prayer may reach deeper levels than usual. You may find yourself with creative insights and a heightened sense of spirituality and enlightenment.

Breaking the juice fast correctly is imperative. On the morning of the fourth day have a juice as your first meal. Midmorning eat an apple. At lunchtime have a detoxifying vegetable juice. Midafternoon have a small bowl of a cooked grain. At dinnertime, have another juice. Then, in the early evening, you can have a small green salad.

The following day you can resume normal eating, but lightly and no toxins. After the three-day fast, refraining from toxins may be much easier than you ever dreamed possible. You'll probably find yourself repelled by toxins and attracted to natural nourishment from the earth and sun.

CHECKLIST FOR THE CLEANSING MONTH

❑ Set up your support system: groups, holistic practitioners, and personal support people.

❑ Review the list of Top Ten Toxins and healthy alternatives. Make a list of your personal toxins and healthier options.

❑ Write down a firm schedule for giving up toxins and a date for juice fasts.

❑ Don't turn to toxins when you're hungry, angry, lonely, tired (HALT), bored, or tense; react with conscious actions and nourishment.

❑ Drink raw juices, including special detoxification juices, throughout the month.

❑ Eat six light meals a day. Drink six to eight glasses of pure water each day.

❑ Take supplements for support on the chemical side. Use herbs, if needed, to facilitate detoxification.

❑ Work with your doctor to reduce or eliminate medications.

❑ If you're unable to give up a toxin on the first attempt or have a relapse, try again.

❑ Go on a one-day raw-juice fast for initial cleansing.

❑ Go on a three-day raw-juice fast to activate your inner healing force.

Good work!

CHAPTER 8

Feel the Force Month: Month Three of the Holistic Self-Health Program

The third month of the program is the time to consolidate your gains and bring all three sides of your Holistic Triangle to new heights of well-being. This month you'll feel the power of your inner healing force and experience higher levels of energy, stamina, and strength.

You'll work and play hard to get closer to your physical ideal and support your evolving body with the healing arts. You'll eat a variety of foods to maximize your energy level and go on a final cleansing fast. You'll experience the synergistic effect of the Holistic Triangle and tap into your innate healing force to overcome lingering ailments.

You'll be revitalized and rejuvenated, generating strength from your empowered Triangle. It's going to be an exciting month!

WEEKS NINE AND TEN

Work Toward Reaching Peak Physical Condition

Lie down, close your eyes, and relax. Visualize how you looked and felt when you were in peak physical condition. Perhaps this was when you were in high school and had all the natural gifts of youth, or maybe it was later, in a period of intense involvement in a sport or exercise program. If you've never been in the best possible shape, imagine how you would look and feel in top condition, and create a clear picture in your mind.

This vision of your optimal physical state is the goal toward which you will be working, both this month and after the program, as you continue your holistic lifestyle.

Take a few minutes to start a new list in your Self-Health Notebook: "Action Plan for Physical Conditioning." Write down all the possible ways you can nourish your physical side to build toward your ideal.

Also, continue to write your Physical and Mental/Spiritual Nourishment reports each day. You should see a rewarding upsurge in your activity and endurance.

Of course, everyone has physical limitations, and you're not expected to become an Olympic swimmer, a prima ballerina, or a basketball star. The holistic goal is to be the best *you* can be; you're not competing against or being compared with anyone else. The emphasis in holistic exercise is always on personal goals, breathing, consistency, and form, not on competition.

Increase the Challenge of Your Exercise Program

During the third month of the program, aerobic exercise should be done at least three times a week, preferably more often, in sessions of at least thirty minutes' duration. The intensity of the workouts can be increased so your exercise pulse is in the high end of your target zone.

Please note: This schedule is based on the assumption you've been following the program up to this point and have been doing aerobic exercise for two months. *If you have not been exercising regularly, you need to go more slowly.* And no matter how high your fitness level, always be conscious of the warning signs of danger during exercise (see page 76). Stop and consult your doctor if you experience any of these signs.

Another goal this month is to increase your stamina and recovery time. How long does it take you to stop feeling exhausted after an aerobic workout? As you get in prime condition, aim to be able to do a specific aerobic exercise for thirty minutes, rest for an hour or two, and then have the energy for a recreational activity, such as a racquet sport or bike riding.

The third month is a terrific time to add variety and challenge to your aerobic program. For example, if you enjoy running, you might want to train for a marathon. If walking is your main exercise, you can try racewalking, walking backward, walking in water, or walking up and down hills.

Your new physical challenge might be an activity you enjoyed in your youth, such as ice skating, jumping rope, ballet classes, or playing on a basketball team. Or it might be a sport that you found appealing but intimidating before: in-line roller skating, skiing, backpacking, snorkeling, or long-distance biking.

Perhaps you'd like to study martial arts, an intense discipline for both the physical and mental/spiritual sides. Iyengar or kundalini yoga classes are also dynamic ways to strengthen the mind/body.

Aerobic dance classes are offered in diverse styles, such as salsa, gospel, Motown, hip-hop, and Broadway jazz. Aqua-aerobic classes, which are given in pools, are great fun and offer the beneficial resistance of water without the impact of gravity.

Step aerobics can be invigorating, provided you don't have a history of knee pain. If you do have weak knees, you may be able to do special therapeutic exercises to strengthen the quadriceps muscles so they support your knees more efficiently. Once you've built these up, you may be able to participate in step classes safely.

Try to get hooked on a form of exercise you thoroughly enjoy. Adults need to have the fun of physicality as part of their lives as much as children do. Find an activity you *want* to do, not one you think you *should* do. Your exercise activity should be a perk, not a chore.

Once you're committed to regular exercise, you may decide to invest in home workout equipment, such as a minitrampoline, treadmill, rowing machine, skiing machine, stair climber, or dual-action exercise bicycle. To get maximum aerobic benefit from exercise bikes and rowing and skiing machines, keep the resistance low so you can go fast, and keep moving for about twenty minutes. Low resistance also reduces the chance of spinal compression and injury. During the last ten minutes of the workout you can increase the resistance to enhance the musculoskeletal benefit.

This is the month to add intensity to your musculoskeletal workout as well as to aerobics. You can increase the number of repetitions of exercises you have been doing steadily, and use small hand weights during your workouts. You might want to work the Nautilus circuit at a gym or purchase weight equipment to use at home. Once you've developed your muscles sufficiently, you might find a sport or exercise class that combines a musculoskeletal and aerobic workout.

Get Expert Support for Your Exercise Program

A book, such as this one, can take you to only a certain point on the physical side. There is no substitute for hands-on training, one-on-one attention, and the personal touch.

This month consider joining a health club where you'll have available the expertise of a personal trainer and a variety of classes. Even if you've joined health clubs before and ended up a dropout, your new strength on the mental/spiritual side might keep you going this time.

If a health club is too expensive or doesn't appeal to you, there are other ways you can learn from the experts without making a major financial investment. Adult schools, community centers, and Y's often have lower-cost programs. Some dance, yoga, and exercise centers allow students to pay on a per-class basis.

Exercise videotapes have the advantage of being relatively inexpensive and accessible at home, but they have two drawbacks.

First, you can develop bad habits and faulty techniques without anyone there to make corrections. Secondly, since there's no one to urge you on, it's easy to quit mid-tape or sit out the harder exercises. For these reasons, exercise videos are best used as a complement to other activities rather than the sole means of fitness.

If you have a program buddy, you can cheer each other on to accomplish your exercise goals this month. If you take a class, you might meet a new exercise friend with whom you can discuss your Self-Health Program and how you're nourishing your physical side. You can also discuss the program with teachers or trainers and ask for their support with your physical goals.

As you rev up your exercise program and transform your physical state, you may experience "growing pains." You may become aware of imbalances, limitations, and conditions that lay dormant when you were less active, and you may suffer joint or muscle soreness or pain.

When your body sends you these messages, it's best to consult a holistic professional, who can tell you if you need to adapt your exercise regimen, who can teach you specific rehabilitative exercises and provide therapeutic treatments. Many holistic chiropractors are experienced in these areas and familiar with sports injuries. Massage therapists can also be skilled in alleviating exercise-related pain.

Give Yourself Extra Physical Nourishment and Care

If possible, treat yourself to at least one professional deep-muscle, full-body massage during the final month of the program. Massage therapy improves circulation and helps disperse fatigue and pain-causing by-products of exercise, such as lactic acid, from the muscles and surrounding tissues.

A session with a talented massage therapist can put you in touch with different areas of your body and let you know where you're holding tension and tightness. This provides insight into how you can warm up more thoroughly before working out and what parts of your body might need continued therapy.

In addition to professional massage, you can exchange massages with your program buddy, friend, spouse, or companion. It's worthwhile reading books on massage or taking a course to learn techniques that are truly therapeutic and not just pleasant. Learning massage together may be a way you can bring your partner into your Self-Health Program and enhance your relationship at the same time. If the best things in life are free, exchanging massages is certainly one of them. You can also use the self-massage techniques on page 226.

The Bathing Ritual in the morning will release muscular tension and start you off in a relaxed mode. But since you're increasing your level of fitness this month, you might need additional hydrotherapy. As you're building muscle, you can use hot and cold compresses to relieve aches and pains and reduce the chance of injury. See page 228 for directions on compress therapy.

If you have an area of achiness resulting from exercise, but no severe pain or injury, you might use a gentle support "sleeve" in the area. Common sleeves include knee supports, elbow supports, ankle supports, wrist supports, or light "corsets" to pull up the abdomen and support the lower back. Use the support only as a temporary measure, until you can build up the weak spot. Continued need for a support indicates you need to learn a healthier technique, reduce the intensity of your activity, or seek professional care.

You can also use natural liniments, such as tiger balm or mineral ice, to relieve achiness and pain. Again, this should be done only on a temporary basis as your body adapts to new demands and growth. If you continue to need any pain relief, consult your holistic doctor.

Stretch, Relax, and Rest

Stretching each day is extremely important when you're doing aggressive aerobics and musculoskeletal exercise. It's vital to keep the joints lubricated, the structure balanced, and the muscles as relaxed as possible.

The bathtub stretches in the morning are a good start, but

don't neglect stretching before and after working out. Too many people are injured because they don't take the time to warm up, cool down, and stay loose. Give yourself the precious gift of ample time for a safe and loving exercise program.

It's beneficial to perform the Total Body Relaxation several times a week this month, especially after cooling down from a strenuous exercise session. Continue practicing deep breathing to increase oxygen intake and stimulate circulation.

A healthy amount of solid sleep is required during this active third month of the program. The additional exercise is likely to help you sleep soundly, but if you do have bouts of insomnia, use the natural techniques on page 90.

Increase Mental/Spiritual Nourishment

Many athletes instinctively use positive visualization to achieve their success. They also channel their belief in their abilities into the discipline and hard practice required for physical excellence. Although you're not expected to become a world-class gymnast or play in the Super Bowl, you can still use the secrets of the stars to attain your personal goals on the physical side of the Triangle.

To use visualization to support your physical development, start by deciding on a specific goal. This may be completing fifty sit-ups and twenty push-ups, keeping up with an advanced aerobics class, or simply swimming continually for thirty minutes—whatever is appropriate for your fitness level and exercise choices.

When you're ready to do the visualization, lie down in a quiet place, close your eyes, breathe deeply, and relax your body. Then see yourself preparing for the physical challenge: putting on your workout clothes, doing a series of stretches, and warming up. Imagine starting the activity, overcoming fatigue and hurdles, and completing what you set out to do. Picture every possible detail: what you're seeing, how your heart is beating, how your body feels, what you hear and smell. Then visualize yourself cooling down, stretching, and feeling triumphant. Keep this feeling in your mind, and try to evoke it several times a day.

Another technique is to lie down and do the Total Body Relaxation exercise. When you are in this receptive state, imagine the sun with all its energy over your head. Feel the energy entering through the top of your head, moving down your face and into your neck. Experience the sun energy filling up your heart and your lungs and being carried by your arteries into your arms and legs. As you breathe, feel vitality flowing in with the oxygen. Focus on the solar energy and oxygen empowering every cell of your body.

When you're fully charged and energized, begin a series of stretches to prepare for your workout. As you stretch, feel the sun energy flowing through your veins. Inhale more power and vitality with every breath. When you're finished with your preliminary stretches, bring this stored energy and power to your aerobic exercise.

While you are exercising, use your mind to maximize the benefits. If you run or walk, visualize yourself moving smoothly and quickly, feeling light and streamlined, taking great strides as if moving on air. If you swim, imagine yourself gliding through the water like a beautiful sailboat on a clear river. When you stretch or do yoga, concentrate on your limbs lengthening, your joints opening up, your body becoming limber and young.

Explore New Varieties of Healthy Foods

This month continue with your Daily Diet Report and healthy eating basics:

- No toxins
- Six small meals a day
- Six to eight glasses of water a day
- Multivitamin/mineral supplements
- At least two raw-juice drinks a day
- A one-day raw-juice fast once during the first two weeks of this month

You may still need to discipline yourself to stay with this nutritional program, but it will probably be much easier than last month. You can make your holistic diet more palatable by trying new varieties of fruits, vegetables, and legumes. Here are some ideas:

—For interesting salads, use arugula, endive, radicchio, mesclun, maché, bibb lettuce, or dandelion greens.

—Add sprouts, lemon grass, chopped nuts, and exotic mushrooms, such as chanterelle or porcini, to salads and other dishes.

—Explore Latin markets for hearty vegetables, such as yuca, plantains, malanga, and boniatos.

—Asian markets are a source of delightful ingredients that can be used in stir-frys and salads: bok choy, Chinese celery, cabbage, water chestnuts, snow peas, wood ears, and fresh tofu.

—Many varieties of squash, including buttercup, calabaza, chayote, delicato, golden nugget, and "spaghetti" squash, can be used for soups and entrées.

—Treat yourself to exotic fruits, such as mangoes, papayas, guavas, kiwis, passion fruit, pomegranates, and star fruit.

This month you might also explore different restaurants where you can stay on your program but enjoy unusual cuisine. Find out if there are any health food or macrobiotic restaurants in your area. Asian, Latin, and nouvelle cuisine restaurants may also have dishes that allow you to stay on the program while experiencing new taste sensations. Just be sure to inquire about ingredients, avoid dishes with too much oil, and ascertain there are no additives, such as MSG.

THE ELEVENTH AND TWELFTH WEEKS

In the final weeks of the program continue with the healthy, high-energy eating pattern, supplements, and lots of raw juices and water for cleansing.

You'll also want to keep up the momentum of your exercise program, with the exception of the fast days. By this time you're likely to be experiencing rewarding improvements on the physical side and a resultant uplift on the mental/spiritual side. Keep going. You're doing great!

Address the Causes of Lingering Maladies

By the last two weeks of the program, many of the conditions and symptoms you had before embarking on the Self-Health journey are likely to be alleviated. If, however, you still have recurrent pain or ailments, this is the time to address these messages.

Write each remaining health problem on the top of a page in your Self-Health Notebook. Research what you can do to correct the root cause of the ailment and prevent it from recurring in the future. Consult books on herbal remedies, foods that heal, vitamin therapy, and body work techniques.

Write down under the symptom all the steps you can take to correct the problem permanently. Also, consult with your holistic doctor to learn what treatment he or she suggests. If you have come across anything interesting in your research, tell your doctor. Remember, you are equal partners, and you may have information your doctor doesn't know.

Once you have written down all the possible solutions, create an action plan. The timetable for this plan may well extend beyond the third month of the program since you may have to counteract years of neglect. But even if you can't overcome your health problems by the end of three months, you can take the primary step: Create a game plan for recovery, and resolve to see it through.

One step you can complete this month is to identify any remaining food intolerances or allergies (see page 194). Most of the common food triggers are eliminated when you give up the Top Ten Toxins; however, it's possible to be allergic to normally healthy foods, and you may need a blood test to track down the culprit.

Allergies to pollen, house-dust mites, animal dander, mold, household chemicals, secondhand smoke, ingredients in cosmetics, and work-related chemicals should also be considered during testing. Once the allergen has been identified, you can take steps to reduce or limit your exposure.

Develop Healthy Posture and Daily Habits

As part of your physical transformation during the final weeks of the program, work on establishing good posture as a permanent habit. Here are some questions that will show you the way to healthy posture:

—When you examine your posture from the side and front while standing:

Is your neck long without being tight (following normal curvature of spine)?
Are your shoulders back instead of rounded?
Is your chest upheld or caved in?
Does your lower back follow the natural spinal curve, or is it flattened or hyperextended (swayback)?
Do you stand tall or lean to one side?

—When sitting:

Do you sit tall, without crossing your legs?
Do you elevate your knees to your hip level or higher (except in a kneeling chair)?

—When sleeping:

Do you have a good, supportive mattress?
Do you sleep with one pillow instead of two?
Do you sleep on your back or side, not your stomach?
Do you keep the window cracked open for ventilation?
Do you rise from bed by turning on your side first rather than using your neck?

—When relaxing:

Do you hold your reading material up to eye level? (If you use bifocals, adjust position so you can maintain posture.)

Do you watch TV from a supportive chair or couch, rather than being propped up with pillows in bed?

Do you frequently get up, stretch, and move around during your leisure time?

—When working:

Do you have an ergonomically designed chair or kneeling chair for work?

Is your keyboard at a comfortable level? Is your computer screen at eye level rather than lower?

Do you hold the phone up with your hand or use a headset instead of jamming the phone between your ear and shoulder?

Do you have fresh air in your office environment?

Do you take stretching breaks at work?

—When walking:

Do you wear comfortable, low-heeled shoes instead of high heels?

Do you look ahead, not down?

—When carrying:

Do you bend your knees and squat before lifting a heavy object?

Do you shift the sides on which you carry objects (or your baby, if you're a parent)?

Do you carry as light a pocketbook as possible and wear the strap diagonally across your chest, or use a lightweight backpack?

You can explore these questions to discover areas of posture and daily habits in which you need improvement. Then write a list of related goals in your Self-Health Notebook. Reading the list several times a day can serve as a reminder. You can also post little notes by your desk, such as "Don't cross your legs!"

As you begin to change your posture, you may experience difficulty or discomfort, since different muscle groups are working. It will take some persistence, but in time your improved postural habits will make you less vulnerable to pain and tension and more confident and attractive.

Continue with Raw-Juice Fasts for Inner Cleansing

During the first two weeks of the final month of the program, it's recommended you go on a one-day juice fast. This will continue the cleansing process and prepare you mentally and physically for a longer fast.

The final raw-juice fast of the program should be planned for the third or fourth week of the month. You can go on a three-day juice fast at this time or a five-day fast. The five-day juice fast is preferable since it allows deeper cleansing of the lymph tissues, liver, and kidneys.

Consult your holistic doctor before going on either fast. Once you have the go-ahead, set your date. Spend two days before the fast eating only fruits and vegetables and drinking juices, herbal teas, and water.

During the three- or five-day juice fast follow all the guidelines beginning on page 188.

There's probably no reason why you can't go to work during the first days of the fast, unless your job is very physically demanding. You just need to plan ahead to have your raw juices available during the workday. If you're lucky enough to have a refrigerator and a relaxed work environment, you can bring your juicer and produce along. Otherwise, prepare the juices in the morning and pack them in thermoses and an insulated picnic bag.

If you're going on a five-day fast, try to have the last two days fall on a weekend.

Be sure to follow carefully the guidelines on page 151 when you break the fast. If you fast for five days, eat lightly for at least forty-eight hours afterward.

Give yourself special treatment during the juice fast. Refrain from strenuous aerobic and musculoskeletal exercise, and concentrate on limbering, deep breathing, and relaxation. If possible, schedule a massage or another therapeutic treatment.

Spend extra time nourishing the mental/spiritual side of your Triangle to get in touch with your higher self during this sensitive period. Take time to listen to your heart, and open yourself up to the endless, infinite love.

Celebrate!

When you've finished the Three-Month Holistic Self-Health Program, plan a celebration. The program has been hard work, and you deserve congratulations and a special treat.

You might want to have a party, as if it were your birthday, only this time you're celebrating feeling younger instead of getting older. The party can be an intimate dinner for you and your love, a small get-together, or a big bash, whatever you please. To mark the occasion with the right spirit, serve natural sun foods and drinks, no toxins. Let your guests know that you're celebrating your self-renewal.

Another way to celebrate completing the program is to take a healthy vacation. This could be a visit to a spa, a spiritual retreat, or a sports-oriented resort. If your funds are limited, take a day trip to a beautiful outdoor spot where you can take a walk, appreciate nature, and refresh your spirit.

You can also celebrate by treating yourself to a professional massage or other body work. You can sign up for a class or buy a piece of exercise equipment to use at home. You can get a new outfit to show off your toned, leaner figure.

For a low-cost celebration, you can give yourself a home spa day. Start with a vigorous workout session, followed by stretching and Total Body Relaxation. Then have a light meal of spa cuisine with a fruit ambrosia drink. You might give yourself a facial with ingredients from your own kitchen and a self-massage with natural lotion. In the evening take a long, hot bath with scented oil and candlelight. Relax and reflect on how much you've achieved during these three months.

CHECKLIST FOR FEEL THE FORCE MONTH

❑ Visualize your peak physical condition, and plan how you can achieve it.

❑ Continue doing aerobic and muscoloskeletal exercise at least three times a week each. Increase the intensity of your workouts.

❑ Try exciting and challenging new forms of exercise.

❑ Seek support and guidance from fitness experts. Consult a holistic health professional to address pain and imbalances, if needed.

❑ Do stretching exercises every day. Do the Total Body Relaxation several times a week.

❑ Support your physical side with creative visualization and affirmations.

❑ Enjoy the benefits of massage. Give yourself compress therapy, if needed.

❑ Eat a light, high-energy diet, drink plenty of water and raw juices, and take supplements. Explore new varieties of wholesome foods. Continue with your Daily Diet Reports.

❑ List all remaining symptoms, and research how to correct and prevent them. Write an action plan for overcoming each problem. Have an allergy test done, if necessary.

❑ Establish healthy posture and daily habits.

❑ Go on a final cleansing juice fast during the third week, for three to five days.

❑ Celebrate the completion of your Holistic Self-Health Program with a special treat.

Congratulations!

CHAPTER 9

Your Healthy Future

The real purpose of attaining better physical health and longer life is not just the enjoyment of a pain- and disease-free existence, but a higher divine purpose for which life was given to us.
—Dr. Paavo Airola

The end of the Three-Month Holistic Self-Health Program is a beginning of your healthy future. The program gave you an opportunity to establish a solid mental/spiritual foundation, detoxify and fortify yourself with healthy foods, and build up your physical side with exercise. Now you have the rest of your life to continue to nourish your Holistic Triangle and love yourself to total well-being.

The primary objective is to incorporate the activities of the program into your permanent lifestyle. It's also desirable to remain in touch with the ever-changing condition and needs of your Holistic Triangle. Nourishing your Triangle is an ongoing, lifelong process, constant yet always changing. The basic forms of nourishment remain the same, but there are different demands and goals as you progress through the years.

EVALUATE YOUR PROGRESS AND ESTABLISH NEW GOALS

A week or two after you have completed the program, retake the evaluation tests in Chapter 5. Compare your scores in each section with the figures from your initial evaluations, taken more than three months ago. It's likely you'll see a dramatic increase in your scores, an upswing that reflects the renewal of your Holistic Triangle.

Of course, the way you *feel* is a more potent reminder of your achievements than any tests can be. The evaluations are only a form of measurement. The reality is your renewed energy, vigor, flexibility, strength, optimism, and empowerment.

However, the tests can help you locate areas of your Triangle that may still need attention and nourishment. Now that you're invigorated, you can tackle these difficult aspects and establish fresh goals.

Write down in your Self-Help Notebook any remaining weaknesses indicated by the evaluations and your own observations. Create a plan for taking healthy action to heal, love, and restore these undernourished areas. Include all the primary and secondary nourishment you can think of that might strengthen these weak links in your Triangle.

You can continue to utilize the evaluations on a yearly basis. Asking yourself these questions each year provides a framework for reflecting on all aspects of your Holistic Triangle. It can help you chart which areas you have been nourishing and which you may have been neglecting. You can use this information to design updated nourishment plans and goals for yourself each year.

EXTEND YOUR MENTAL/SPIRITUAL STRENGTH

Now that you've learned the art of loving yourself to health, it's an excellent time to share the wealth. Extend your love, energy, and knowledge to people who need your help.

You might want to introduce the ideas of holistic health to your family and friends, in a loving, nonjudgmental way. Once they've seen your transformation, they may be more open to the concepts than they were initially.

If you're eager to have your family make healthy changes, such as giving up toxins or exercising more often, take a positive approach, rather than a negative judgmental stance. Let them know how much healthier you are now that you've detoxified, how much happier you feel now that you're in touch with your spirituality, how much you enjoy being fit. Present holistic activities as being fun and rewarding, rather than as something they *should* do.

If the people you love are not ready to make major changes, encourage them to take small steps in the right direction. But if they are completely resistant and unwilling to change, you may have to accept their attitude. No one can be responsible for another person's Triangle. All you can do is set a good example and keep on loving others unconditionally.

If anyone you know is inspired by your example to go on the program, you can volunteer to be her or his buddy and support throughout the three months. You can offer to refer the person to holistic health professionals, share your books and information, and be his or her exercise partner. But be sure you *offer* rather than *force* your advice and participation. The Self-Health Program is a personal journey, and everyone has her or his own way.

You can also share your mental/spiritual energy by doing volunteer work. Pick a group of people for whom you feel genuine compassion, and volunteer to assist on a regular basis, whether it's once a month or once a week.

When you can care for people who are very different in circumstances, yet understand they are basically the same inside, your spiritual side grows enlightened. You learn the meaning of unconditional love on a spiritual, rather than merely intellectual, level. And the more you reach out, the more you tap into the infinite love in the Universe.

When you're helping less fortunate people, remember, we all have the same basic needs. Not everyone is ready to understand or accept the concept of the Holistic Triangle, but every person on the planet needs to nourish his or her mental/spiritual, chemical, and physical sides. And we all need more unconditional love and acceptance. Now that you've been consciously nurturing these qualities within yourself, you are in a powerful position to share your love with others.

Another way to share your mental/spiritual empowerment is to become active in your community or in a national group. For example, you might organize a health food co-op in your town or work toward creating a new park. On a national or global level, you can volunteer for an environmental group or lobby the government to reform the health care system. There are so many ways in which you can make a difference in the world, with faith and action.

LIFESTYLE CHANGES

The period of peak condition after the program can be an optimal time to undertake necessary lifestyle changes involving your relationships, home, or career. These may be changes you have wanted to make for a long time, or they may be an outgrowth of your higher level of awareness.

Remember, however, that any change is stressful, and it's best not to undertake too much at once. Pace your progression realistically, with patience, acceptance, and self-consideration. Don't initiate so many sudden changes that you find yourself unable to keep nourishing your Triangle.

Loving Relationships

The first part of your lifestyle you may want to consider concerns intimate relationships. If you are involved with a person who is abusive, self-destructive, highly critical, negative, or withholding, this will inevitably undermine your mental/spiritual base. This erosion is likely to lead to weakness on the chemical and physical sides and eventually harm your health.

The period following completion of the Self-Health Program, when you feel empowered and capable of change, may be a good time to deal with an unhappy relationship. This may mean seeking help from a psychotherapist, family counselor, spiritual leader, substance abuse program, or support group.

Ultimately, if your partner refuses to seek help or change behavior that is hurting you both, you may need to leave the relationship. A crucial part of loving yourself is the ability to disengage from a person who is unable to receive and reciprocate your love.

Your Holistic Triangle can give you precious support when you're dealing with a painful relationship. Your mental/spiritual foundation of unconditional self-love provides the strength to take action. Faith and spirituality offer profound comfort. Wholesome, balanced nourishment on the chemical side supplies energy and helps prevent stress-related illness. On the physical side, exercise releases uplifting hormones, releases tension, and feeds self-esteem. The Bathing Ritual, Healing Moments, and relaxation sessions are also soothing support when you are dealing with stressful personal issues.

Nourishing Work

Work is another aspect of your lifestyle to examine after the program, when you are feeling confident and clear.

It's natural for human beings to have a degree of resistance to hard work, but it's not healthy to dread your job every day. A certain amount of pressure is unavoidable in the workplace, but a high level of stress on a long-standing basis will wear down your Triangle.

Perhaps you need to work on changing your *attitude* toward work. We can't always control what happens to us, but we can usually control how we react. Control doesn't mean repression; the goal is to maintain a sense of perspective and balance in your reactions and to avoid the physical effects of stress.

Affirmations, visualizations, deep breathing, and meditation can help you learn not to overreact to the demands of your job. Biofeedback training, meditation, relaxation practices, and yoga can reduce the stress response. There are also books and courses offering stress reduction techniques specifically for the workplace.

If an unfair boss or unpleasant coworker causes you to dislike your job, you may be able to use your mental/spiritual power to rise above that person's level and refuse to be provoked. Remind yourself that his or her negativity is a symptom of mental/spiritual weakness and lack of self-love. *Your* self-love is unconditional and does not depend on anyone's approval.

If you find your work boring or demeaning, try to find ways to make it more challenging. Many managers are impressed when employees offer to take on new responsibilities or carry the job a step further than required, and this can lead to a more rewarding position.

If you try different approaches and still find your work extremely stressful, upsetting, boring, or unsatisfying, you may need to move on. Or you may be unwillingly forced into a period of unemployment at some point in your career.

Whatever the circumstances, your Holistic Triangle can help you during a job search. On the mental/spiritual side, faith, self-esteem, and such techniques as creative visualization and affirmation are supportive. On the chemical side, a nourishing diet provides stamina and reduces the chance of illness during a stressful job hunt. On the physical side, a toned, fit appearance fosters a positive first impression during interviews. You can rally all three sides of your Triangle to help you get the job you deserve.

A Healing Home

The third major aspect of your lifestyle to consider when you are planning a healthy future involves your home. Is it a sanctuary? Is it conducive to relaxing and replenishing your Triangle? If not, what can you do to make it a more peaceful, serene, comfortable place?

Some people are able to create sanctuaries for themselves in apartments in the middle of cities. They thrive on the diverse people, stimulating culture, and high-powered jobs in the urban environment. Other people find cities depleting and need daily contact with nature to stay sane and de-stressed.

Look into your heart and ask yourself what you need. Don't be afraid to ask if your environment is healthy for your spiritual as well as physical state. Do you have easy access to forms of exercise you enjoy? Do you feel safe and comfortable in your area? Do you have people you know and care about nearby?

When you've thought about these questions, you may discover that you're fine where you are or learn you would be happier in a different environment. Moving to a healthier location may be a long-range goal, requiring years of planning, saving, and hard work. But once you decide on a plan and make a commitment, you're on your way.

CONTINUE TO NOURISH YOUR MENTAL/ SPIRITUAL SIDE

Many people continue to work out and maintain healthy diets after the three months of the program but start to neglect the mental/spiritual sides. This is often the first part of the Triangle to be ignored, yet it is the most sustaining.

Many aspects of spirituality and holistic health have been touched upon in this book. Why don't you choose a practice or topic that piques your interest and delve into it more deeply?

For example, if you're attracted to meditation, you can read books by the masters, take classes, or practice with a spiritual group. If you found affirmation and visualization useful, you can read more, listen to tapes, go to seminars and workshops, and practice, practice, practice.

If you're intrigued by herbal healing, you can read up on the subject or study with an herbologist. Perhaps you'd enjoy a vegetarian cooking course or like to learn about the healing qualities of different foods.

These are just a few examples. The potential for learning and strengthening the mental/spiritual side is truly infinite. And you can expand this side for the rest of your life. Although a certain amount of decline on the physical side is inevitable, your mind can continue to flower.

CONTINUE TO NOURISH YOUR CHEMICAL SIDE

On the chemical side of the Triangle, the basic goal after the Self-Health Program is to adopt healthy eating as a way of life. As you get older, it becomes more and more crucial to eat light, wholesome food, avoid toxins, and take supplements. A young person's chemical side can take a lot of abuse, but as the years go by, you need to be careful.

You may be able to indulge in toxins occasionally if you're strong and well. But it's safer not to begin to think of these indulgences as "treats," or you may end up treating yourself to an early grave.

When you take a toxin, think about why you did it. Remember the triggers—hunger, anger, loneliness, tiredness, boredom, and tension—as well as societal influences. Refresh your knowledge of alternative ways to deal with these emotions as well as healthy substitutes for the toxin itself.

If you find yourself craving a certain toxin, reread the reasons why it is detrimental to your health. Remind yourself that you stopped before, during the program, and you can stop again. You don't have to be a slave to any food, drink, or chemical. You're free, and you love yourself enough to make healthy choices.

One of the healthiest choices you can make is to continue raw-juice fasting on a regular basis. Raw-juice fasting one day a week is highly beneficial for inner cleansing and rejuvenation. Think of the raw-juice fast as a weekly Sabbath for your body, a spiritual and chemical day of rest.

It's also an excellent practice to go on a three- to five-day juice fast four times a year. This will allow you to rest and renew your internal environment on a seasonal basis, as nature renews itself.

Drinking plenty of water each day and eating small frequent meals of plant foods are also healthy habits to maintain. Taking vitamin and mineral supplements each day will benefit your immune system and help keep you well.

CONTINUE TO NOURISH YOUR PHYSICAL SIDE

If you want to feel youthful and energetic, continuing your regular exercise program is a requirement. Exercise is a key to maintaining optimism, confidence, and a zest for life. It is also essential for reducing your chance of suffering from heart disease and other leading causes of early death.

Try to do some type of physical activity on a daily basis. Unless serious conditions interfere, you should be able to exercise for the rest of your life. The intensity of exercise does, however, need to be modified in later years. Stretching can continue to be a daily routine and can stave off the symptoms of aging.

Other forms of physical nourishment are also lifetime companions: plenty of sleep, deep breathing, relaxation practices, massage, and the Bathing Ritual. If you find yourself neglecting your physical side because you're "too busy," plan a day off to give yourself a home spa treatment.

Since we're all subject to the effects of gravity, stress, and aging, body work is recommended on an ongoing basis, not only when you have pain. Chiropractic adjustments can help prevent osteoarthritis, painful trigger points, and fibrous lesions from developing. Other secondary forms of physical nourishment, such as massage treatments, are also nourishing. Try to have some preventive, therapeutic body work at least once a season.

It's also a fine idea to stay in touch with your holistic doctor, even when you're feeling good. By having regular checkups, you can obtain an objective assessment of your condition and become aware of any developing problems. You can also discuss new research findings, family illnesses, and other concerns that crop up. Your holistic doctor can get to know you on a personal basis and have greater insight into what you need to do to keep your Triangle vital and balanced.

DEALING WITH SETBACKS

When most people finish the Three-Month Holistic Self-Health Program, they feel so terrific they plan to continue their healthy lifestyles forever. But as the weeks, months, or years pass, they find it easy to slip into old habits. A cup of coffee once in a while becomes a cup every morning, then two a day, until it's back to four cups a day. They figure dessert once in a while won't hurt and soon crave sugar after every meal. They decide to skip an aerobic walk because it's rainy one day, the next day they're tired, and soon exercise is no longer a habit.

The human ability to make excuses and rationalizations is limitless. You need to be careful not to fool yourself into believing you can neglect your Holistic Triangle and not suffer the consequences. If you're not totally honest with yourself, you can get trapped in a system of self-delusion and denial.

If you decide to have a nitrate-loaded hero sandwich, a cola, and a slice of cream pie for lunch, fine. Just be honest and tell yourself: I'm choosing to eat something that will weaken my Holistic Triangle, and I'm going to end up feeling worse. If you tell yourself it doesn't matter, today's special treat can easily become tomorrow's unhealthy habit.

Being a holistic person certainly doesn't mean you'll never taste a toxin again for the rest of your life. There are special occasions when it's appropriate to break the rules. If you've been nourishing your Triangle conscientiously, your body can handle the toxins, for a short time. But it's a fine line between "once in a while" and every day, a line that can creep up on you. You don't have to be fanatical, but you have to be vigilant. *You* are the only person who can guard your precious well-being.

The danger of relapses is they can be self-perpetuating. The most common pattern is the following: You start eating foods that cause blood sugar imbalance and don't supply wholesome nourishment. Your energy level drops, and you stop exercising regularly. You gain weight, and old symptoms return. You feel ashamed and stop loving yourself.

There are many other reasons why people turn away from a

holistic lifestyle. Unfortunate events or negative influences can undermine their mental/spiritual foundations, leading to neglect of the other sides of their Triangles. Illness or injury can cause people to lose faith in their innate healing power, and they stop making self-health efforts.

Life is a constant pull between dark and light, negative and positive. No one's perfect, and it's easy to fall into a downward slide. If you find this happening, it's time for drastic action. It's time to commit to three months of self-renewal and go on the Holistic Self-Health Program again.

The program is not meant to be a once-in-a-lifetime experience; it's meant to be a lifelong tool. Use it when you feel addiction creeping up on you; when you feel depressed, stressed, or fatigued; when you have persistent health problems; or whenever you need rejuvenation.

A LIFELONG COMMITMENT

In a way, loving yourself to health is like a happy marriage. You start off with the Self-Health Program, which, like a wedding, is a rite of passage. It takes a lot of preparation and effort, but you remember it for the rest of your life. After the ceremony you're full of hope and optimism. But as time passes, you learn it requires a lot of love, caring, attention, compromise, and effort to keep it going.

As the years go by, you have your ups and downs and plateaus. But if the commitment and faith and unconditional love are there, the holistic lifestyle will see you through.

No one is immune to the whims of fate, and no one lives forever. But you do have a great deal of control over the *quality* of your life. By nourishing each side of your Triangle, you can give yourself the ultimate gift: a positive, high-quality life.

CHECKLIST FOR YOUR HEALTHY FUTURE

❑ Retake the Self-Health Evaluations. Write down areas of weakness and an action plan for more nourishment. Continue using the evaluations as a learning tool periodically.

❑ Introduce friends and family to holistic health ideas. Help them make positive changes if they are ready.

❑ Do volunteer work on a regular basis.

❑ Undertake necessary lifestyle changes involving your relationships, your home, and your career. Pace yourself carefully; don't take on too many stressful changes at once.

❑ Continue to nourish your mental/spiritual side by delving more deeply into areas of interest.

❑ Continue to nourish your chemical side by avoiding toxins, enjoying plenty of wholesome foods, drinking water, and taking supplements. Continue raw-juice fasting on a regular basis.

❑ Make a holistic exercise routine a permanent part of your daily life.

❑ Continue to do the Bathing Ritual, and practice deep breathing and relaxation techniques. Replenish your Triangle with sufficient sleep.

❑ Have secondary forms of physical nourishment, such as chiropractic care and massage, on a regular basis.

❑ Be totally honest with yourself. Don't let rationalizations cause you to abandon healthy habits.

❑ If you find yourself in a downward cycle, embark on the Three-Month Holistic Self-Health Program again.

❑ Make a lifelong commitment to nourish your Triangle and give yourself plenty of love.

PART THREE

SELF-HEALTH RESOURCES

CHAPTER 10

Self-Health Resources:
The Mental/Spiritual Side

GUIDELINES FOR MEDITATION

1. Meditate in a quiet place where you won't be disturbed. Sit cross-legged on the floor if you're comfortable in this position, or sit upright in a chair. (You may want to do the Total Body Relaxation on page 218 or some stretching exercises to relax your body before meditating.)
2. Close your eyes. Establish a deep breathing pattern: Breathe slowly, through your nose if possible, into the abdomen, ribs, and chest. Exhale slowly and completely.
3. You can either focus on your breath or concentrate on a focal word. "Om" is an ancient and universal mantra. You may prefer "one," "peace," or "love"; a brief phrase such as "let go" or "good health"; or the Sanskrit mantra *om shanti* or *ham sah*. Repeat your mantra silently in sync with your

breathing as you inhale and exhale. Try to keep your thoughts only on the focus word and your breath.

4. When your mind wanders, quietly bring your thoughts back to your breath and your focus word. It will become easier to remain focused with practice. Try to practice once a day for ten to twenty minutes. You may want to set a timer when you start, so you aren't tempted to check the clock.

5. Allow yourself a few minutes after meditation to sit quietly and breathe; then rise slowly and stretch before resuming your activities.

NOTE: Meditation can cause anxiety initially since it can be disturbing to be left alone with your mind. Observe the anxiety, and carry on without judging or allowing fear to take control.

Meditation is a way to learn to observe your mind more objectively, without letting emotions take the upper hand. In a sense, it's paradoxical since meditation gives you more control over your mind and also teaches you to let go.

GUIDED HEALING VISUALIZATIONS

Basic Healing Session

Lie down on the floor, and begin slow, deep breathing. Relax each part of your body, starting with your feet, up through your calves, your buttocks, your abdomen. Relax your spine along the floor, all the way up through the back of your neck. Let your body sink into the floor, and relax.

Now focus on the part of your body where there is pain or illness. Look inside, and see what the malady is trying to tell you. What are you doing or not doing that may be causing the imbalance in your body? What organ or system has been neglected or abused and is now manifesting itself in a symptom? How can you give yourself more nourishment in that area?

Tell the part of your body that is in pain or dysfunction it is part of the whole and you love it. Even if you can get no message about what action to take to heal yourself, send your unconditional love to the area that is symptomatic.

Tell the symptom that you are going to take action to heal it. Imagine yourself taking this action. Inhale the love and healing power of the Universe. Send it to the part of your body that is in pain. You can visualize this healing power as a warm white light. Feel it melt and dissolve the discomfort. Enjoy the soothing, healing nourishment you take in with every inhalation.

Picture yourself in glowing good health. Think of yourself getting up, going through your day, and the next, in superb condition. Stay with these images until they are firmly established in your mind.

Before rising from this healing session, stretch your arms overhead, lengthening your body along the floor. Then slowly move to one side, and get up gently.

Immunity Visualization

Lie down, and begin with deep breathing and the body relaxation, as in the previous visualization.

Picture your white blood cells, the janitors inside your body, which clean up toxins. Imagine these cells gobbling up toxins and harmful bacteria. See the white blood cells engulf and digest the debris, consuming it and rendering it harmless.

Visualize your bloodstream as being clean and clear, flowing freely, without obstruction or pollution. The white blood cells have swept away disease-causing poisons, and your system is strong and healthy.

Visualization to Alleviate Back Pain

(Before you do this visualization for the first time, it is helpful to look at the drawing of a spine on page 92 so you can picture the vertebrae in an aligned state.)

Begin by lying down and breathing deeply into your abdomen. The cleansing breath flows up your spine, nourishing and lengthening it. As you inhale, the breath brings energy up your spine. As you exhale, the vertebrae relax and elongate, relieving pressure on the nerves. Take time to focus on each area of your spine. Wherever there is tightness and constriction, send this area your breath until it releases the tension.

When your spine feels comfortable, focus on the muscles of your back, and pinpoint the painful area. Visualize these muscles as knotted, frayed rope. Slowly concentrate on unknotting the rope. Smooth and stretch it out. Then do the same to the parallel muscles on the other side of your spine. Feel the muscles unknot until they are long and smooth and your back is free.

CHAPTER 11

Self-Health Resources: The Chemical Side

HEALTHFUL MEAL PLAN GUIDELINES

1. Breakfast: When you first wake up, have a glass of water, warm water and lemon, or herbal tea. After your bath, enjoy one or two of the following:

   Fresh fruit
   Whole grain cereal with soy milk
   Whole grain pancake
   Whole grain toast with nut or fruit butter

2. Midmorning snack: A midmorning snack can help you avoid a slump and the urge for caffeine. Try one of these choices:

   Fruit

A small portion of nuts or seeds
A protein drink made with a natural supplement powder
Raw vegetable or fruit juice

3. Lunch: Lunch should be your biggest meal of the day since this is when your body is producing more enzymes and you have the most activity ahead. Some options:
    Green salad
    Raw or steamed vegetables
    Cooked legumes and grains
    Seeds and nuts
    Fish

4. Midafternoon snack: Give yourself a treat:
    Fruit, seed, and nut mix
    Almond milk or soy beverage
    Fresh fruit
    Fruit-sweetened whole grain baked goods

5. Dinner: This meal is interchangeable with lunch, although it's best to eat smaller portions than earlier in the day. Also, it's recommended to eat dinner as early as possible:
    Green salad
    Raw or steamed vegetables
    Cooked legumes and grains
    Seeds and nuts
    Fish

6. Evening snack: A light bite an hour or two after dinner:
    Fruit
    Crudité with healthy dip
    Raw fruit or vegetable juice from your juicer

RAW-JUICE FASTING

To understand why raw-juice fasting is so effective, it helps to realize that the gastrointestinal (GI) tract, from the mouth to the anus, is actually one big juice extractor. The purpose and function of the GI tract are to break down complex foods into simple ones that can be assimilated.

Raw-juice fasting allows us to rest the often overworked GI tract. The juicer does much of the work the gastrointestinal tract normally does; it separates the liquid from the fiber and the nutrients from the pulp.

While juice fasting has dramatic effects, it is not a miracle cure or a quick fix. The primary step toward nourishing the chemical side of your Triangle is to decrease or eliminate toxic input and increase healthy input. After you have made some progress in reducing toxic input, you can consider a one-day juice fast.

Not only is raw-juice fasting a detoxification tool, but raw juices are a wonderful addition to your daily diet. The juices provide the essential nutrients of fruits and vegetables in a concentrated form that is easily absorbed.

Raw juices provide high levels of antioxidants, which can provide protection against cancer, heart disease, and the aging process. Antioxidants protect against free radicals (molecules containing a highly reactive unpaired electron) and pro-oxidants (molecules that promote oxidative damage). While these molecules are naturally produced in our bodies, environmental factors contribute to their proliferation. Free radicals can bind to and destroy other cellular components, and have been linked to the development of chronic degenerative diseases.

To counteract these degenerative disease-promoting agents, we need nutritional support. Our cells can protect us against free radical and oxidative damage with the help of antioxidants and enzymes such as carotenes, flavonoids, vitamins C and E, and sulfur-containing compounds.

Raw juice is far superior to canned, bottled, or frozen juice because it contains more of these vitamins and enzymes. Packaged juices are pasteurized, a process that causes the loss of many vitamins and minerals as well as the life force itself.

Raw juicers are an essential health appliance, since they separate the liquid from the pulp, while blenders merely liquefy everything. It pays to invest in a high-quality, high-performance juicer that will last.

If you purchase your juicer at a health food store, you can also get a book on juicing, with recipes and recommendations on which fruits and vegetables are helpful for specific conditions. Juicing can be used as targeted therapy as well as an overall preventive.

It also pays to buy organic produce to use for your raw-juice fasting. The Environmental Protection Agency has identified sixty-four pesticides as potential cancer-causing compounds, and you don't want to risk ingesting these chemicals in your raw juice, particularly when fasting. If you cannot obtain organic produce, clean your produce with a biodegradable rinse, available in health food stores. Even organic produce should be washed carefully before juicing, then cut into small pieces.

Follow the directions that come with your juicer, or obtain a guide to juicing for specific directions for all produce. Here are some of the fruits, vegetables, and combinations you can use:

- Apples, alone or with apricots, berries, grapes, lemons, pears, oranges, kiwis, papayas, peaches
- Bananas, alone or with cantaloupes, mangoes, oranges, papayas
- Berries, alone or with oranges, pears, apples
- Cherries, alone or with pears, peaches, pineapples
- Grapefruit, alone or with oranges, papayas, pineapples
- Grapes, alone or with lemons and apples
- Lemons and limes, in combination with sweet fruits
- Mangoes and papayas, alone or with oranges, pineapples, bananas
- Oranges, alone or with papayas, peaches, bananas
- Pineapples, mixed with berries or oranges
- Plums and prunes
- Watermelon, alone or with other melons

- Asparagus and green beans, added to carrots and apples
- Beets, with carrots, spinach, sweet potatoes, parsley, celery
- Broccoli, with carrots, celery, parsley
- Cabbage family vegetables (cabbage, broccoli, cauliflower, brussels sprouts, kale, collard, radishes, turnips), mixed with carrots, celery, parsley

- Carrots, alone or in combination with virtually all other vegetables
- Celery, alone or in combination with cucumbers, parsley, kale, spinach, fennel, lettuce
- Dandelion root, mixed with fennel
- Garlic and ginger, added to vegetable combinations
- Lettuce, added to carrots and celery
- Onions, added to carrots and parsley
- Parsley, added to carrots, cucumbers, other vegetables
- Peppers, with tomatoes
- Potatoes, added to carrots and other vegetable juices
- Spinach, with tomatoes, beets, carrots, parsley, cucumbers
- Tomatoes, alone or with cucumbers, parsley, watercress, spinach, peppers

DETOXIFICATION RECIPES

The following recipes are especially created to promote detoxification during the Self-Health Program. Drink the raw juices slowly, and stop when you are satisfied. Depending on your size, an adequate serving may be from six to twelve ounces.

Some of these concoctions don't taste delicious, but that doesn't mean you shouldn't drink them. As part of the program, you need to satisfy all the organs of your body, not just your taste buds. Instead of fixating on the flavor, concentrate on how the juices purify and strengthen your body. But if you simply can't bear the taste of a vegetable juice, add some apple or pineapple. All fruits and vegetables should be washed carefully and scrubbed, but do not peel unless specified.

Love Your Lungs Juice

---

6 carrots (with tops cut off)
Large handful of spinach
4 sprigs watercress
Large handful of parsley
¼ peeled potato

Love Your Liver Juice

---

3 apples* (chopped into quarters or wedges with seeds removed)
2 carrots (with tops removed)
1 beet
1 cucumber (waxed cucumbers only should be peeled)
*People undergoing sugar withdrawal should use green apples.

Fresh Skin Tonic

---

2 apples (chopped into wedges with seeds removed)
1 cucumber (waxed cucumbers only should be peeled)
2 slices pineapple* (with skin removed)
½ lemon* (peeled)
*People with citrus allergies or skin problems should substitute kale or parsley for lemon and pineapple.

Immune Booster Drink

---

4 carrots (with tops removed)
3 stalks celery (bottoms removed)
Handful of lettuce (any type except iceberg)
Small piece gingerroot (optional)

Vascular Rejuvenator

4 carrots (tops removed)
3 stalks celery (bottoms removed)
Handful of kale
Handful of spinach
Handful of alfalfa sprouts
Dash of cayenne pepper

Detoxification Special

3 carrots (tops removed)
2 beets
2 stalks celery (bottoms removed)
½ cabbage
½ white potato
¼ onion (peeled)
½ clove garlic (peeled)
Sprinkle of ginger

When you're in the mood for a warm beverage, try this vegetable broth, which is high in minerals and serves as an alkalizer:

Vegetable Broth

3 potatoes, chopped
3 carrots (tops removed)
3 stalks celery (bottoms removed)
1 beet
1 turnip
2 cloves garlic, chopped
½ onion, peeled & chopped
Seasoning to taste

Add all ingredients to two quarts of water. Bring to boil, lower heat, and simmer for ½ hour. Strain out vegetables, and let broth cool to warm temperature.

NOTE: To turn this into a *Fiber Broth* that relieves constipation, add 2 tablespoons flaxseed or bran. Refrigerate the broth overnight; then heat and drink it in the morning.

FOOD SENSITIVITIES

Food allergies and food intolerance can cause many different immunological and physiological responses and symptoms. These can include:

—Headache, migraine, fatigue, faintness, depression, anxiety, hyperactivity in children, blurred vision, dizziness, difficulty concentrating
—Sinusitis, rhinitis, earache, ear infection
—Cramps, vomiting, nausea, stomach ulcers, duodenal ulcers, diarrhea, irritable bowel syndrome, constipation, wind, bloating
—Water retention, vaginal discharge, frequent urination
—Joint pain, rheumatoid arthritis, muscle aches, weakness
—Rapid pulse
—Hives, eczema, swelling

While these symptoms *may* be caused by food sensitivities, they may also have other bases. It takes detective work to determine if a food is the allergen, and if so, which substance.

Many of the Top Ten Toxins are common culprits in food sensitivities. These include milk and other dairy products, chocolate, coffee, beef, and food additives. If you eliminate these toxins, you may automatically overcome food reactions.

However, a food sensitivity can also result from an inappropriate immunological response to a normally healthy substance. Healthy foods that cause reactions in some people include wheat, citrus fruits, corn, nuts, potatoes, soybeans, tomatoes, and spices.

There are several ways to track down food allergies:

Elimination diets: This involves avoiding suspected allergens for two weeks. Then you reintroduce the suspects one at a time, waiting several days to see if any symptoms arise. The problem with this method is it requires a great deal of patience and can be inexact and confusing.

The pulse test: This self-test is sometimes, but not always, effective for detecting food sensitivities. Find a place under your wrist where you can feel your pulse. Sit quietly, and relax for a minute. Count your pulse for sixty seconds to determine your resting pulse. Eat just one of the foods you suspect is an allergen, without eating anything else. Test your pulse thirty minutes later, then sixty minutes later, also while resting. If your pulse is twenty or more beats higher than the first resting pulse, this food may be an allergen. Stop eating the food for two weeks, and see if your symptoms are alleviated.

Direct blood test: The blood test for allergies involves an initial drawing of blood in a doctor's office. This is then sent to a laboratory for comprehensive allergy testing. This method is highly effective, although not foolproof.

The skin prick test: Also done in a doctor's office, this tests how the skin reacts to a range of common allergens. A prick or scratch is made in the skin, and a minute amount of an allergen extract is allowed to enter it. This can result in a reaction known as the weal-and-flare response. Skin prick tests are efficient for identifying inhaled allergies, but often fail to detect food allergies.

Once the allergen is identified, there are several treatment options. The treatments to avoid are allergy shots, which are based on the vaccination theory and consist of injections of small doses of the allergen. While this may give you temporary relief, it can lead to the development of an allergy to another substance or a worsened reaction when you discontinue the shots. Allergy shots insult the body's innate wisdom and, like most quick fixes, can backfire.

A safer option is simply to stop consuming the food to which you are allergic. In the case of many foods, after the initial withdrawal period you can easily do without it for the rest of your life.

If, however, the allergen is a healthy food, such as wheat, you can reintroduce it after you have been through the Self-Health

Program. Then watch yourself carefully to see if reactions occur. Some people overcome allergies to inherently healthy substances by ridding their bodies of accumulated toxins and building up their immune systems. Detoxification can also result in reduction or disappearance of allergies to inhalants such as pollen.

SUPPLEMENTS

The Food and Drug Administration has mandated that manufacturers cannot advertise the superiority of vitamins from natural food sources over synthetic vitamins. However, saying there is no difference between these two types is like saying there's no difference between coal and diamonds. They both derive from carbon, but one form is obviously superior.

Synthetic vitamins are artificially produced in laboratories. Natural vitamins are derived from living food sources. Which do you think would contain more easily assimilable nutrients?

The most important supplement for all of us is a high-quality multivitamin/mineral. When you're choosing your multisupplement, look for a natural product with a comprehensive range of vitamins and minerals. Unless this is a time-released product, it's recommended to take it several times a day, so there is a constant flow of nutrients into your system.

There are also special supplements that are useful to take on a periodic basis in addition to vitamins and minerals. These include kelp, brewer's yeast, spirulina, chlorella, acidophilus, rutin, lysine, and royal bee's jelly.

As well as provide a backbone of basic strength and strong immunity, supplements can be used for specific therapeutic purposes. The chart at the end of this chapter will give you more information about the specific properties of different vitamins and minerals.

The Required Daily Allowance (RDA) provides, in many cases, a minimal amount of supplementation. If you want to give the chemical side of your Holistic Triangle maximum nourishment, you can double the amount of many vitamins and minerals to provide the Optimum Daily Allowance (ODA).

VITAMINS

Vitamin	Function	Natural/Organic Source	Deficiency Condition	Excess Condition	Depleted by	Caution	RDA (ODA approx. twice RDA)
A carotenoids	Enhances immunity; antioxidant; aids in cancer prevention; needed for skin repair and maintenance plus bone and tooth formation; required for protein synthesis.	Alfalfa, apricots, asparagus, beets, broccoli, cantaloupes, carrots, fish liver oil, liver, garlic, kale, papayas, parsley, peaches, red peppers, sweet potatoes, spinach, yellow squash, turnip greens	Dry skin, itchy eyes, sensitivity to light, night blindness, influenza, and infections	Nausea, headaches, aching bones, hair loss, and irritability	Exposure to strong light, pollution, certain medications, drugs	Individuals with liver disease, diabetes, and hypothyroidism should consult a physician before taking large doses	5,000 IU 50,000 or more can be toxic
B₁ thiamine	Beneficial to circulation, blood formation, learning capacity, muscle tone for heart, intestines, and stomach muscles; aid to hydrochloric acid production and carbohydrate metabolism	Dried beans, brown rice, liver, peanuts, peas, rice bran, soybeans, wheat germ, brussels sprouts, oatmeal, plums, prunes, raisins, egg yolks, fish	Forgetfulness, fatigue, beriberi, insomnia, digestive problems, muscle tenderness; possible weight loss	Rapid or irregular heartbeat, restlessness, trembling, low blood pressure, cold sores, edema	Alcohol, tobacco, drugs, sugar, baking soda, overcooking food sources of B₁; also antibiotics and oral contraceptives	A diet high in carbohydrates increases the demand for thiamine	1.5 mg
B₂ riboflavin	Required for formation of red blood cells, cell respiration, growth, and metabolism of carbohydrates, fats, and proteins; facilitates oxygen use in skin, hair, and nails; vitamin A and B₆ maintain mucous membranes in digestive tract	Beans, cheese, eggs, fish, poultry, spinach, yogurt; also asparagus, avocados, broccoli, brussels sprouts, nuts	Eye fatigue, cracks and sores in the mouth, dandruff, carpal tunnel syndrome, purple tongue	Itching, tingling in arms and legs	Light, cooking, antibiotics, alcohol, drugs	Oral contraceptives and strenuous exercise increase the demand for riboflavin	1.8 mg
B₃ niacin, niacinamide, nicotinic acid	Supports nervous system, circulation, healthy skin; lowers cholesterol; also used to treat mental illnesses; helps prevent plaque formation in arteries	Beef, fish, broccoli, carrots, potatoes, tomatoes, corn flour, whole wheat, cheese, eggs; also tuna, halibut, and swordfish	Dermatitis, depression, diarrhea, pellagra, loss of appetite	Results in niacin flush; antidote: two large glasses of water	Emotional stress, drugs, cooking	High amounts contraindicated for pregnancy, diabetes, gout, liver disease, ulcers, glaucoma, hypertension	20 mg

Vitamin	Function	Natural/Organic Source	Deficiency Condition	Excess Condition	Depleted by	Caution	RDA (ODA approx. twice RDA)
B₅ pantothenic acid	Required by all cells of body, especially organs; aids in production of adrenal hormones and antibodies; necessary for steroid and cortisone production in the adrenal gland	Beans, beef, eggs, saltwater fish, mother's milk, whole wheat, fresh vegetables, yeast, wheat germ, peanuts	Depression, fatigue, poor coordination, heart trouble, headache, cramps	Not yet determined	Drugs and alcohol, stress	No known side effects	2 mg
B₆ pyridoxine	Affects physical and mental functions of body; helps maintain balance of sodium and potassium in body; required for normal brain function, nervous system, RNA and DNA synthesis; reduces symptoms of premenstrual syndrome; natural diuretic	Carrots, spinach, peas, eggs, fish, brewers' yeast, sunflower seeds, walnuts, wheat germ. Less rich sources of pyridoxine; avocados, bananas, beans, blackstrap molasses, cabbage, cantaloupe, pears	Anemia, diarrhea, skin and mouth disorders, convulsions, blindness, loss of appetite	Not yet determined	Oral contraceptives, cooking and soaking food, drugs	Antidepressants, estrogen, and oral contraceptives deplete the body of pyridoxine	2 mg
B₁₂ cyanocobalamin	Required to prevent anemia, for digestion, absorption, protein synthesis, carbohydrate and fat metabolism; prevents nerve damage; maintains fertility; promotes normal growth	Mostly found in animal sources; lamb, beef, crabs, clams, herring, liver, mackerel, seafood; also eggs, almonds, cheese, tofu, most grains	Malabsorption, which is common in the elderly; blood disorders, hardening of the arteries, fatigue, pernicious anemia, memory loss, hallucinations, abnormal gait	High hemoglobin count	Drugs, stress, history of ulcers, gastritis	Vegetarians need to supplement their diet with B₁₂ since it is found mostly in animal products	3 mcg
Biotin also known as vitamin H for hair growth	Aids in cell growth, healthy hair, skin, sweat glands, nerve tissue, bone marrow; required for metabolism of carbohydrates, fats, and protein	Most foods, especially peanuts, beans, egg yolks, oyster, saltwater fish, poultry, soybeans	Deficiency is rare because biotin is produced naturally in intestines; absorption problems would cause fatigue and/or depression	Not yet determined	Antibiotics, sulfa drugs, which destroy intestinal flora that normally produce biotin	Raw egg whites contain a protein called ovadin that combines with biotin and depletes the body of this vitamin	Not yet established

Vitamin	Function	Natural/Organic Source	Deficiency Condition	Excess Condition	Depleted by	Caution	RDA (ODA approx. twice RDA)
Choline	Required for nerve transmission, gallbladder regulation, liver function; reduces buildup of excess fat in liver	Egg yolks, legumes, liver, meat, whole grains	Brain function and memory impairment; fatty acid buildup in the liver, cirrhosis of liver	Not yet determined	Drugs and alcohol, stress	Not established	Not established
Folic acid	Formation of red blood cells, DNA synthesis; cell division and reproduction of cells; regulates embryonic and fetal development of nerve cells	Barley, beans, lentils, navy beans, beef, bran, brewers' yeast, brown rice, cheese, chicken, dates, green leafy vegetables, split peas, root vegetables; salmon, tuna, wheat germ, whole grains	Abnormally red tongue, low white blood cell count; depression, brain damage, nervousness, anemia	Not yet determined	Drugs, oral contraceptives, stress	Avoid large dosages if you have experienced convulsions or have a hormone-related cancer	1–2 mg
Inositol	Hair growth, lecithin formation, fat and cholesterol metabolism; aids in prevention of hardening of arteries	Fruits, vegetables, whole grains, yeast	Not yet determined	Not yet determined	Large amounts of caffeine	Not established	Not established
PABA (para-aminobenzoic acid)	Protects against sunburn and skin cancer; is an antioxidant; assists in formation of red blood cells	Liver, yeast, brown rice, molasses, whole grains	Loss of hair color (graying of hair may be restored if caused by nutritional deficiency or stress), fatigue, depression, constipation, headaches	Suspected in topical skin disorders	Sulfa drugs	Not established	Not established
C ascorbic acid, mineral polyascorbate, (nonacidic buffered)	Beneficial as antioxidant especially when combined with vitamin E; promotes tissue growth, repair; enhances immunity; prevents bruising; heals wounds. Polyascorbate is more efficient form of C.	Citrus fruits, berries, green vegetables, asparagus, avocados, beet greens, broccoli, cantaloupe, mangoes, onions, papayas, parsley, green peas, sweet peppers, spinach, rose hips, tomatoes, turnip greens	Easy bruising; lowered resistance to infection, colds, and flu; tooth decay; gum disease; thyroid insufficiency; premature aging; anemic; deterioration of collagen	Diarrhea; lower dosage gradually until bowel can tolerate vitamin C level	Aspirin, alcohol, analgesics, oral contraceptives, steroids, antidepressants	Pregnant women should not use more than 5,000 mg per day	60 mg ODA 1–3g

Vitamin	Function	Natural/Organic Source	Deficiency Condition	Excess Condition	Depleted by	Caution	RDA (ODA approx. twice RDA)
D calciferol, ergosterol, viosterol Sunshine vitamin	Assimilates calcium, phosphorus, and other minerals within digestive tract; important for growth and development of bones and teeth in children	Fish-liver oils, fatty saltwater fish, eggs, sprouted seeds, mushrooms, sunflower seeds, sweet potatoes, vegetable oils; also sunlight when absorbed in the skin	Rickets, tooth decay, pyorrhea, osteomalacia, osteoporosis, poor bone and growth in children, premature aging	Excessive doses can can be toxic over a period of years; 65,000 IU or more synthetic D3 not recommended	Antacids, mineral oil, cortisone, and some cholesterol-lowering drugs	Vitamin D should not be taken without calcium; synthetic D may cause abnormal calcium deposits	5–10 mcg Sunshine is best source (not between 11:00 A.M.–1:00 P.M.; avoid burning)
E tocopherol	Effective antioxidant, preventing cancer and cardiovascular disease; promotes healing of wounds, normal blood clotting; aids in prevention of leg cramps and cataracts; required for healthy reproductive organs	Cold pressed vegetable oils, nuts, seeds, sprouted seeds, whole wheat, fresh wheat germ, green leafy vegetables, legumes, eggs, brown rice, cornmeal, oatmeal, sweet potatoes; Alpha is best (fat-soluble)	Heart disease, sexual impotency, reproductive disorders, miscarriages, muscular disorders	Not yet determined	Not yet determined	Diabetics and those suffering from rheumatic heart disease, an overactive thyroid, or hypertension should use small dosages	8–10 IU ODA 400 IU
F	Lowers blood cholesterol; required for healthy skin and mucous membranes; helps body utilize calcium and phosphorus	Cold pressed vegetable oils; most abundant in soybean, sunflower, safflower, and flaxseed oils	Skin disorders—eczema, dandruff—hair loss, prostate, menstrual, and kidney disorder	Not yet determined	Stress	No known problems; must have essential fatty acids	Not established
K	Necessary for normal blood clotting; converts glucose to glycogen, which affects liver	Kelp, alfalfa, brocoli, soybean oil, egg yolks; also brussels sprouts, blackstrap molasses	Hemorrhages, nosebleeds; premature aging	Flushing, sweating	Antibiotics hinder absorption; interferes with anticoagulants	Large doses can can be toxic to newborn; heart disease	Not established
Bioflavonoids citrin, hesperidin, quercitin, rutin	Not a true vitamin; assists in the absorption of vitamin C; strengthens capillary walls; acts as anticoagulant; promotes circulation; reduces cholesterol; helps treatment of cataracts	Fresh fruits, particularly pulp: grapes, apricots, strawberries, black currants; cherries; also prunes, buckwheat	Hemorrhoids, varicose veins, bleeding gums, eczema, psoriasis, hemorrhages, radiation sickness, coronary thrombosis, atherosclerosis	Diarrhea	Cooking	No known documentation	Not established

MINERALS

Mineral	Function	Natural/Organic Source	Deficiency Condition	Excess Condition	Depleted by	Caution	RDA (ODA approx. twice RDA)
Boron	Works with calcium to develop and maintain healthy bones	Green leafy vegetables, fruits, nuts, and grains	Few people deficient in boron	Not yet determined	Not yet determined	3 mg per day maximum	Not yet determined
Calcium	Required for development and maintenance of bones and teeth; beneficial to heart and nervous system; prevents cramps; aids in normal blood clotting	Dairy products, dark leafy vegetables, sesame seeds, sardines, seafood, almonds, dandelion greens, figs, filberts, tofu, turnip greens, organic nonpasteurized goat's milk, fortified nut milk	Osteomalacia, osteoporosis, depression, brittle cracked nails, muscle cramps and spasms, tooth decay, eczema, hypertension, sore joints	Hinders absorption of zinc	Antacid tablets taken as a source of calcium which interferes with absorption; heavy exercise, sugar, high-protein and fat diets	Do not take supplements if suffering from kidney disease or kidney stones	800–1,200 mg
Chlorine	Aids liver in detoxifying body; helps produce hydrochloric acid in stomach, required for protein and mineral assimilation	Kelp, seaweed, kale, saltwater fish, avocado, chard, tomatoes, cabbage, endive, celery, cucumber, asparagus, oats	Poor digestion; imbalance of fluid levels in the body	Not documented	Stress	Highly toxic in large doses; avoid heavily chlorinated pools	500 mg
Chromium	Removes glucose from blood to produce energy; maintains blood sugar levels; synthesizes heart protein	Brewers' yeast, naturally mineralized water, corn and corn oil, whole grains, nonalcoholic beer	Diabetes, hypoglycemia, atherosclerosis, heart disease	Not yet determined	Refined white sugar	Not determined	Not established ODA 100 mcg
Cobalt	Required for synthesis of vitamin B_{12}; also hemoglobin formation	Green leafy vegetables	Pernicious anemia	Not documented	Stress		Not established
Copper	Production of RNA facilitates healing; required for the absorption of iron; maintains natural color of hair and skin; benefits nervous system	Almonds, avocados, barley, beans, green leafy vegetables, mushrooms, pecans, soybeans	Anemia, loss of hair and hair color, heart damage	Depletes vitamin C and zinc	Excess amounts of zinc and vitamin C	Not determined	2–3 mg

Mineral	Function	Natural/Organic Source	Deficiency Condition	Excess Condition	Depleted by	Caution	RDA (ODA approx. twice RDA)
Fluorine	Utilized in development of healthy bones and teeth; acts as antiseptic; prevents infections	Sunflower seeds, cheese, garlic, beet tops, green vegetables, almonds	Not known	Can be toxic, stains teeth	Not known		Not established
Iodine	Highly beneficial to thyroid gland, physical and mental development	Kelp, seaweed, dulse, Swiss chard, saltwater fish; garlic, pears, pineapple, artichokes, egg yolks	Enlarged thyroid, fatigue, lethargy, loss of interest in sex, possible mental retardation and breast cancer	Metallic taste and sores in mouth	Raw and excessive amounts of cabbage, cauliflower, kale, which interfere with absorption	Limit iodine in the diet if a hypothyroid condition exists	0.15 mg
Iron	Most important is production of hemoglobin, which carries oxygen from lungs to red blood cells; beneficial to immune system and normal growth patterns	Eggs, fish, liver, blackstrap molasses, prunes, raisins, brewers' yeast, spinach, turnip greens, sesame seeds, beets and beet tops, sunflower seeds	Anemia, hair loss, brittle nails, fatigue, dizziness, lightheadedness, shortness of breath on exertion, headaches	Hemochromatosis, cirrhosis, diabetes, possible heart disorders; link to cancer	Coffee and tea interfere with absorption; excessive perspiration	Zinc and vitamin E inhibit absorption; excess amounts also produce free radicals	Males 10 mg Females 18 mg
Lithium	Metabolizes sodium beneficial to nervous system, particularly involuntary nerves	Kelp, seawater	Nervous and mental disorders	Not known	Stress	Used for bipolar mental disorders; must be monitored	Not established
Magnesium	Important in enzyme activity; required for healthy muscles and bones; acts as tranquilizer	Nuts, green leafy vegetables, fish, seafood, soybeans, kale, endive, figs, apples, blackstrap molasses, brown rice	Kidney damage, muscle cramps, nervousness, depression, twitching	Not known	Alcohol, caffeine, diarrhea, diuretics	Competes with calcium for absorption; use separately Balance 1:1 ratio	350–400 mg
Manganese	Protein and fat metabolism; fat digestion; benefits nervous and immune system; coordinates action and communication between brain, nerves, and muscles; aids in production of breast milk	Avocados, nuts, green leafy vegetables, spinach, beets, seaweed, kelp, apricots	Impeded growth, sterility, poor equilibrium, asthma, tinnitus	Not known	Stress	No known side effects	Not established

Mineral	Function	Natural/Organic Source	Deficiency Condition	Excess Condition	Depleted by	Caution	RDA (ODA approx. twice RDA)
Molybdenum	Nitrogen and carbohydrate metabolism	Whole grains, brown rice, millet, buckwheat, brewers' yeast, dark green leafy vegetables	Mouth and gum disease, gout, sexual disorders in male	Interferes with copper metabolism	Stress	Only small amounts needed	Not established
Phosphorus	Bone and teeth development healthy nervous system and mental activity; heart contraction	Most foods contain some phosphorus: whole grains, seeds, nuts, legumes, egg yolks, apricots, avocados	Poor nerve and brain function, poor sexual performance, lack of strength, lack of energy	Interferes with calcium absorption			Adults 800–1,200 mg Children 1,000–1,400 mg
Potassium	Required for proper muscle contraction, for maintaining proper acid-alkaline balance; maintains blood pressure and prevents stroke	Bananas, potatoes and potato peels, apricots, blackstrap molasses, brewers' yeast	Severe deficiency will allow salt to accumulate in the body; damage to heart; hypertension; disorders of nervous system		Stress, diuretics, diarrhea	Muscle weakness from high intake	1,875–5,625 mg
Selenium	Important antioxidant; protects immune system; works with vitamin E to produce antibodies; helps restore liver after damage	Brewers' yeast, Brazil nuts, broccoli, mushrooms, most vegetables depending on soil content they are grown in	Muscle deterioration, liver damage, premature aging, intestinal and colon cancer	Not known	Stress	Only small amounts needed	Not established
Silicon (silica)	Necessary for healthy hair, skin, and nails; forms collagen, which connects bones	Alfalfa, flaxseed, oats, apples, grapes, beets, onions	Brittle nails, hair loss, poor bone growth, Alzheimer's disease	Not established	Stress	Only small amounts needed	Not established
Sodium	Maintains proper body fluids, electrolyte balance; required for hydrochloric acid production in stomach	Kelp, seaweed, sea salt, celery, asparagus	Dehydration, heart palpitations, confusion, low blood sugar	High blood pressure, water retention, stomach ulcers and cancer, heart disease	Excessive perspiration, diarrhea	Excessive sodium is common in junk foods, lunch meats, antacids	200–600 mg

Mineral	Function	Natural/Organic Source	Deficiency Condition	Excess Condition	Depleted by	Caution	RDA (ODA approx. twice RDA)
Sulfur	Important for healthy hair, skin, and nails; disinfects blood; stimulates bile secretion; slows down aging process, synthesizes collagen, which keeps skin moist	Radish, turnips, onions, kale, cabbage, eggs, garlic, brussels sprouts	Poor skin tone, eczema, brittle nails, dull hair	Flatulence	Moisture and heat	Avoid hard-boiled eggs	Not established
Zinc	Has great importance to healthy prostate and reproductive organs; beneficial to immune system and formation of RNA and DNA; aids in elimination of toxic carbon dioxide	Fish, seafood, green leafy vegetables, pumpkin and sunflower seeds, brewers' yeast, egg yolks, lima beans	Birth defects, poor growth development, enlarged prostate, loss of sexual function	Daily doses of 100 mg or more inhibit the immune system	Diarrhea, diabetes, kidney disease, cirrhosis of liver	See excess condition	15 mg

HERBS

Herbs can be used in many ways, including:

—Compresses: Cloths soaked in herb solutions are applied to areas that need healing.

—Essential oils: Oils are distilled from herbs and used externally or in the form of inhalants or teas.

—Extracts: These very effective forms for healing are usually taken orally.

—Ointments and salves: Generally used for bruises, sores, and inflammations, these are applied externally.

—Poultices: Moistened, hot herbs are spread on cloths and applied to areas of body to relieve pain and inflammation.

—Powders: Herbs are ground into powders, often used in capsule or tablet form for specific disorders.

—Tinctures: Powdered herbs are added to a solution of alcohol and water.

The seeds, stems, roots, bark, leaves, and flowers of hundreds of different plants are used as herbal remedies. Here is an introduction to a dozen helpful herbs and some of their benefits.

Herbs	*Uses*
Alfalfa	Helps detoxify the body and promote pituitary gland function. Helpful for arthritis, anemia, colon disorders, diabetes, and ulcers.
Capsicum (Cayenne)	Improves circulation and aids digestion. Good for kidneys, lungs, pancreas, heart, and stomach.
Catnip	Aids digestion, helps relieve stress, and can control fever. Good for colic, colds, flu, inflammation, and pain.
Chamomile	Aids digestion and stimulates appetite; used as a nerve tonic and sleep aid. Helps relieve blad-

der problems, colds, fever, headaches, colitis, hemorrhoids, muscle cramps, and pain.

Comfrey root
: A blood cleanser; good for stomach, kidneys, bowels, and lungs. Helps coughs, ulcers, swelling, cramps, pain, and burns.
CAUTION: Should be used only under the supervision of a health professional.

Echinacea
: Has antibiotic, antiviral, and anti-inflammatory properties. Helps the immune system and lymphatic system and is used for colds, flu, and infections.

Garlic
: Detoxifies the body and protects from infection; strengthens blood vessels and can lower blood pressure.

Goldenseal
: A natural antibiotic that detoxifies the body and strengthens the immune system. Benefits the heart, liver, spleen, pancreas, and colon. Useful for colds, flu, diabetes, hypoglycemia, and inflammation.

Lobelia
: Acts as a cough suppressant; can reduce fever and cold symptoms. Good for sore throats, laryngitis, bronchitis, and colds.

Parsley
: Benefits thyroid, lung, stomach, bladder, liver, and kidney function. Helps goiter, obesity, fluid retention, indigestion, gas, and menstrual disorders.

Pau d'arco
: A natural antibacterial agent; has a healing and blood-cleansing effect. Good for infection, diabetes, ulcers, allergies, candidiasis, and immune dysfunction diseases.

Peppermint
: As a digestive aid helps control diarrhea, spasms, and indigestion. Can also relieve sinus problems and headaches.

NATURAL ALTERNATIVES TO COMMON NONPRESCRIPTION DRUGS

Painkillers

If you frequently take aspirin, acetominophen, or ibuprofen to overcome pain, you need to work with your health care professional to ascertain the root cause of the pain. Then you can decide on a treatment plan to correct the problem and prevent it from recurring.

This treatment may include dietary changes, therapeutic exercise, chiropractic care, physical therapy, massage, relaxation techniques, biofeedback, or acupuncture. Giving up toxins alone may alleviate your recurrent pain, but you may also need expert assistance.

Cold and Sinus Medicines

If you often resort to drugstore cold and sinus remedies, try the following alternatives.

- Eliminate toxins, especially dairy products.
- Drink powdered, buffered vitamin C in juice and water throughout the day.
- Drink eight glasses of water a day.
- Drink peppermint and other herbal teas, with lemon and a little honey.
- Take garlic in capsule form and in food.
- Take herbal supplements of echinacea and goldenseal.

Laxatives

If you take pharmaceutical laxatives, you can adopt healthier ways to avoid constipation.

- Eliminate dairy products, meat, white flour, and sugar, which contain no fiber.
- Drink eight glasses of water a day.
- Eat more high-fiber foods: beans, peas, fresh vegetables, fresh fruit, whole grains, and such dried fruit as figs and prunes.
- Add bran or flaxseed to cereal, juices, or the Fiber Broth recipe on page 193.
- Exercise is another way to relieve constipation without the artificial stimulation of laxatives.

SUPPLEMENTS TO AID DETOXIFICATION

During the Self-Health Program it is recommended that you work with a holistic professional to establish a vitamin/mineral/ herbal supplementation program tailored to your particular condition and needs. However, if you are unable to set up a customized supplementation program, here are some general guidelines:

Take a high-quality, time-release multivitamin/mineral supplement after breakfast and after dinner.

Take a B complex supplement after your midmorning and your midafternoon snacks.

Take a buffered, esterized form of vitamin C three times daily as a detoxifier, for a total of one to three grams, depending on your size. If you experience diarrhea, cut down the dosage until you reach a tolerance level.

Take a multiplex amino acid blend after dinner.

Chromium, also called GTF (glucose tolerance factor), is a mineral that works with insulin in the metabolism of sugar and is required during withdrawal from hypoglycemic-related toxins, such as sugar, alcohol, and caffeine. Check your multivitamin/ mineral supplement, and if it does not contain this mineral, purchase a chromium supplement and take one hundred micrograms daily.

Add a teaspoon of spirulina powder to two of your raw juice drinks each day, or take two spirulina tablets after two meals. Spirulina is high in protein, vitamins, and minerals and also has chlorophyll for cleansing.

Valerian, which is available in capsule form, can be used occasionally for its calming effect, particularly when overcoming an alcohol or drug addiction. *Do not use valerian for prolonged periods of time.*

Chamomile is a gentle sedative for the mind and body that also helps with indigestion that may arise during detoxification. You can prepare the flowers in tea form and drink a half cup at a time. Do not use chamomile if you are allergic to ragweed.

Catnip tea can also soothe the nerves. Alfalfa tea is rich in vitamins and minerals and acts as a cleanser. Pau d'arco tea and a mixture of echinacea and goldenseal tea are effective detoxifiers and may help strengthen the immune system. Other teas you can use intermittently include rose hips, dandelion, and red clover.

CHAPTER 12

Self-Health Resources: The Physical Side

MONITORING YOUR PULSE DURING WORKOUTS

During your aerobic workout you need to monitor your pulse rate. Here is the formula for establishing the target zone of your exercise pulse rate:

220 minus your age, multiplied by 0.60 = low end of target rate

220 minus your age, multiplied by 0.80 = high end of target rate

For example, if you are thirty-four years old, you would calculate this way: $220 - 34 = 186 \times 0.60 = 111.6$ low end

$$220 - 34 = 186 \times 0.80 = 148.8 \text{ high end}$$

Your target zone would be 111 to 148 heartbeats per minute during exercise.

If you have not been doing aerobic exercise on a regular basis before starting the Self-Health Program, the intensity of your workout should be in the low end of your target zone. For example, if you're thirty-four, during the first few weeks you should aim for an exercise pulse rate of 111 to 120 beats per minute. By the end of the program you might work up to an exercise pulse rate of 130 beats per minute.

You can take your pulse either in the soft area of the wrist, just under your thumb, or at the carotid artery at the neck. Unless you are elderly, the carotid pulse may be easier to count during exercise. You can take the carotid pulse on either side of your windpipe, to the right or left of the Adam's apple area.

About five minutes into the aerobic exercise session, place your finger (not thumb) gently on the pulse and count the beats for fifteen seconds, then multiply by four to get your exercise pulse rate. If it is too high up in your target zone or above the zone, you need to reduce the intensity of the exercise. Do this test again near the end of your aerobic sessions.

If all this pulse arithmetic sounds too complicated, there is an alternative. Sporting goods stores offer a device called the pulsemeter to wear on your wrist. You put in the parameters, and the meter beeps when your pulse is too high or too low. It's also a handy device for tracking your progress from workout to workout.

MUSCULOSKELETAL DEVELOPMENT EXERCISES

Here is a simple set of musculoskeletal development exercises that focuses on the muscle groups that are generally the weakest. You'll recognize some of the basic exercises of gym classes and calisthenics, but with an emphasis on proper form and breathing.

Breathing is primary in a holistic approach to exercise. The exercise rate should be directly connected to a comfortable respiratory rate. The rule is: Exhale on exertion; inhale on relaxation of movement.

These exercises should be done in comfortable, flexible clothing and supportive workout footwear. Work out on a carpet or, preferably, an exercise mat. An exercise mat is a good investment since you can also use it for your stretching exercises. *Always do some gentle stretches before the musculoskeletal sequence.*

Leg Raises

These are intended to strengthen the abdominal group of muscles. Leg raises also tone and strengthen the leg and buttocks muscles.

Lie on your back with your left knee bent and left foot flat on the floor; right leg stretched out. Place your hands under your lower back. You might also place a small folded towel under your lower back for more support.

IMPORTANT NOTE: Keep your lower back on the floor during all leg raises, and consciously use your abdominal muscles. If you let your lower back arch, you risk injury and are not properly working the abs.

1. Exhale as you lift your right leg about six inches off the ground. Breathe and hold the leg up until you feel fatigue. Inhale as you lower slowly. Repeat on the left side (with right leg bent and right foot on floor).
2. Exhale and raise your right leg slightly higher. Hold it up; breathe; lower slowly. Repeat on left side.
3. Exhale and raise your right leg to a forty-five-degree angle, parallel to the bent left leg. Hold it up; breathe; lower slowly. Repeat on the left.
4. Exhale and raise your right leg six inches off the floor *to the side.* Hold it up; breathe; lower slowly. Repeat on left.
5. Exhale and raise your right leg slightly higher, to the side. Hold it up; breathe; lower slowly. Repeat on left side.
6. Exhale and raise your right leg to a forty-five-degree angle, as high as the bent leg, to the side. Hold it up; breathe; lower slowly. Repeat to the left.

The goal is to do this six-part set three times on each side. However, if you haven't been training, start off with one set, and work your way up to more repetitions.

As you strengthen the abdominals, you can add clockwise and counterclockwise leg circles, always with the nonworking leg bent in and the foot on the floor. Later you can add ankle weights to the exercise.

Sit-ups

Sit-ups will strengthen the abdominal muscles, but remember, we want to do sit-ups, not "neck-ups." Concentrate on using your abdominal muscles and not straining your neck. Depending on your fitness level, you may be able to rise only an inch off the floor using just your abs. That is fine. When you're stronger, you can rise halfway up and increase the number of repetitions.

Bend both knees, feet on the floor. Place your feet under a piece of furniture or have someone hold them steady. Bend your elbows, and place your thumbs under your ears, index fingers on top of your ears. Keep your elbows to the side; don't use them to get up. You can also do sit-ups with your arms straight out in front of you.

Exhale and sit up, only as far as you can go using your abdominal muscles. Inhale through your nose as you lower your body to the floor. Repeat at least ten times to start. Add repetitions as you build up your abdominal muscles.

If you cannot rise at all with your hands in the suggested position, cross your arms diagonally across your chest. This reduces the body weight and makes sit-ups easier.

After you have worked out for a period of time and can do up to thirty sit-ups, rising halfway up, you can begin diagonal sit-ups, rotating toward the opposite knee. Be careful with rotation; don't rotate too far or rise up too high.

Push-ups

These develop the upper back, shoulder, and arm muscles as well as strengthen the abdominals.

Lie on your stomach, and place your hands slightly wider than your shoulders and your feet close together. Keep your legs and body in a straight line as you push up. Don't let your back arch or your pelvis drop; your body must be kept in a straight line to prevent injury and work the upper muscles.

Inhale deeply; then exhale as you push up, keeping your body straight. Inhale as you lower your chest to the floor; exhale as you push up. Repeat as many times as you can while maintaining proper form, without getting shaky.

Many women find they cannot do even one push-up when they begin training. If this is your situation, you can do modified push-ups, with your knees bent and lower legs on the floor. This reduces the weight you need to push up, until you can build up strength and do full push-ups. Be very careful not to flex your lower back in the modified push-up position, and place padding under your knees if needed.

Buttocks Exercises

These are often called doggie exercises since they're done on all fours, an undignified but effective position.

1. Position yourself on your hands and knees, back straight (except for the natural curve of the spine). Exhale and lift your leg to the side, keeping your knee slightly bent. Inhale and lower. Repeat ten times on each side. As your buttocks muscles get stronger, work up to three repetitions of ten on each side.
2. On all fours, inhale and bring your knee into your chest and your chin down, rounding your back. Exhale and bring your leg back, as you lift your head and slightly arch your back. Repeat ten times on each side. Move slowly, with attention to form and breathing. This exercise works the upper body muscles as well as the buttocks and provides a nice stretch for the neck.

Jumping Jacks

These are intended to build muscular and cardiovascular endurance. Jumping jacks work the muscles of the legs, arms, and chest, develop coordination, and are a good lead-in to aerobic exercise. If you do your jumping jacks in front of the mirror, you can check on the synchronicity of your arms and legs.

Supportive footwear is required for this exercise. If you have arthritis, lower back pain, or joint weaknesses or are elderly, jumping jacks are not recommended.

Start with your feet together, arms at your side. Inhale, then exhale as you bring your arms overhead and open your legs. Inhale as you bring your feet together and arms down. Repeat ten to fifty times.

As you develop endurance, you can do quadrant jumping jacks: Jump a quarter turn to the right side, then to the back, to the left side, and front.

STRETCHING SEQUENCE

Here is a stretching sequence that lasts about thirty minutes. It provides a good overall stretch that will relax you after a hard day of work or prepare you for aerobic exercise.

1. Lie down on your back, and breathe deeply into your abdomen.
2. Lift your arms over your head, and keep them on the floor. Slowly stretch your right arm and right leg, lengthening the whole right side; then release. Stretch and lengthen your left arm and leg; then release. Stretch and lengthen both arms and legs; then release. Repeat this sequence once.
3. Bend both knees, and place your feet flat on the floor, with your arms out to the sides. Lengthen your spine along the floor. Slowly drop your knees to the right side, looking left. Breathe in this position. Bring the knees center; then drop slowly to the left side, looking right. Return to center, and repeat.
4. Lie with your arms out to the sides, legs down. Bend in the right knee. Cross it over to the left side, looking and twisting your upper body to the right, to form a diagonal oppo-

sition stretch. Breathe in this position. Slowly return to center. Stretch your leg up in the air; then bring it down. Bend in your left knee. Cross it over to the right, while stretching your upper body and head to the left. Breathe; then return to center, stretch your leg up, and bring it down slowly.

5. Hug your knees into your chest, tuck in your head, and rock up to a sitting position. Sit in a comfortable cross-legged position. (If it's difficult for you to sit cross-legged, you can do these head and neck exercises from a standing position.) Be very gentle with the neck movements.

6. Slowly turn your head right to left, four times. Lower your chin to your chest. Then slowly raise your head into an arching position. Whenever you arch, think of lengthening your neck up, rather than back. (Don't drop your head all the way back and compress your neck.) Lift up and down four times. Then stretch your neck diagonally by dropping your ear toward your shoulder (although it won't touch), twice to each side. Do two slow head circles to the right; two slow circles to the left. Again, don't let your neck drop back.

7. After the head movements, if you have been sitting cross-legged, stretch your legs in front, and place the leg that was underneath before on top as you resume cross-legged position. Lift your shoulders up; then relax them, four times. Bring your shoulders into your chest; then stretch them toward the back, four times. Circle your shoulders to the back four times and to the front four times. Place your hands on your shoulders, and circle your elbows to the front four times and back four times.

8. With your knees bent, roll down slowly; then turn onto your stomach. Stretch your right leg up about six inches off the ground, hold for a few breaths, and lower. Stretch your left leg up, hold, lower. Stretch both legs up; hold while you breathe, and lower. Relax your legs.

9. Return to a sitting position, legs stretched out in front. Stretch your arms overhead; then reach forward over your legs. Keep your chin up and your back long as you grab

your legs and stretch forward. Don't pull or round your back; keep a slight arch in your lower back, and breathe into the stretch. Then roll up slowly, and shake your legs gently.

10. Bend in your knees so your feet are touching. Stretch forward between your legs, keeping your chin up and your back elongated. You can also stretch first toward one knee, then the other in this position. With your knees bent, roll down slowly.

11. Turn onto your stomach. Place your hands, elbows bent, about six inches outside your shoulders. Inhale and slowly lift your head, then slowly arch your spine. Use mainly your torso strength, not your hands, to rise. Keep your elbows slightly bent, and don't compress your lower back in the arch. Breathe for several counts; then lower slowly.

12. Staying on your stomach, bend your knees and clasp your ankles. Slowly lift your upper body and legs into a bow position. Hold for a few counts as you breathe, then lower slowly and relax. (You may need to exercise regularly for several weeks before you can do this "bow" exercise.)

13. Turn onto your side, and then rise to a standing position gently. Lift up tall through your spine. Keeping your hips front, slowly twist your upper body to the right and wrap your arms around your waist, looking right. Breathe in this position; then unwrap and shift to center. Repeat to the left side.

14. Place your feet a few feet apart. Keeping your hips forward, stretch your left arm overhead and tilt your body slightly to the right. Return to center. Stretch your right arm overhead and upper body to the left. Return to center.

15. Bring your feet back under your hips. Slowly roll down, starting with your head, rolling down one vertebra at a time, bending your knees slightly as you lower. Hang and relax; then roll up slowly, starting with the bottom of your spine and your head coming up last. Repeat the rolling up and down once.

16. Stand tall, feeling your posture and alignment. Imagine light and energy flowing all the way up your spine, up into

your head. Try to keep this feeling as you start your aerobic exercise or go about your day.

TOTAL BODY RELAXATION

Find a quiet, private room, and lower the lights. Lie down on a padded surface, but not a bed since you don't want to fall asleep.

Begin deep breathing. Fill up your abdomen, rib cage, and lungs with healing breath. Exhale slowly, and let your body sink into the floor. Feel the support of the earth. Let your body release and relax with every exhalation. Continue deep breathing as you focus your relaxation on the different parts of your body.

Relax your toes. Relax the soles of your feet. Let your heels sink into the ground and relax.

Relax your calves. Let them feel very loose and long. Relax your thighs. Let your thighs soften and relax. Your legs are long and relaxed.

Relax your hips. Feel them wide and relaxed. Let your buttocks sink into the ground and relax.

Relax your abdomen. Feel the breath relaxing and nourishing your organs. Your organs are relaxed and functioning smoothly.

Relax your rib cage and chest. Feel it open and relaxed.

Relax the base of your spine. Feel the relaxation flowing up your spine with your breath. Feel your lower back soften and relax. Let your middle back relax.

Feel your shoulder blades wide and relaxed on the floor. Let your upper back relax and release. Your spine is long; your muscles are released; your back is completely relaxed.

Feel the relaxing energy enter your fingertips. Relax your lower arms, your elbows, your upper arms. Let the relaxation flow into your shoulders. Relax the tops of your shoulders.

Let the relaxation flow up your neck. Let your head sink into the floor, supported by the earth. Your neck and your head are completely relaxed.

Relax your jaw. Relax your mouth. Relax your cheeks. Relax behind your ears. Relax your eyes. Relax your forehead. Your face is completely soft and relaxed.

Your entire body is relaxed, from your toes up through your legs, your organs, your back, your shoulders, your neck, your face.

Every breath you take is full of love. Feel the love flowing to all the open, relaxed parts of your body.

Meditate on the love flowing freely throughout your body.

When you are ready, open your eyes, and gently stretch. Roll onto one side, and rise slowly.

THE BATHING RITUAL

The following bathing sequence is called the Bathing Ritual because it provides spiritual as well as physical nourishment. If you do it regularly, it will become an integral part of your life and provide precious comfort and pleasure.

The best time to do the Bathing Ritual is in the morning, as a way to start your day by nourishing your Holistic Triangle. The bathing sequence takes only about fifteen minutes, and the benefits are well worth your getting up a little earlier. Try it and you'll see.

Set the scene by having a clean bathtub and natural light, if possible. You can use a scented candle, potpourri, or aromatherapy oils to enhance the atmosphere if you wish.

1. Fill the bathtub approximately one-quarter full with hot water, as hot as you can comfortably tolerate. The water level should be shallow enough so that you can lie with your back on the bottom of the tub, neck relaxed, and only your face above water.
2. Step in slowly, and sit down, feeling the heat relax each part of your body. Then slide down slowly until the back of your head is underwater (your head may rest on the bottom of the tub or float an inch or so). Bend your knees,

and rest your feet against the wall at the opposite end of the tub or up on the sides.

3. Breathe deeply through your nose, and say a positive affirmation to yourself, such as "My mind and body are calm and relaxed." Relax and let your body melt into the warmth.

4. With your arms alongside your body, tilt your right ear toward your right shoulder, keeping the left shoulder down, to stretch your neck laterally. Hold for five seconds; then return to center. Repeat toward the left side.

5. Bring your chin and your chest up slightly to arch your head back. Hold for five seconds; then shift your head slightly to the right and left in the arched position. Return to center.

6. Inhale, hold your nose, and turn your head to the right. Hold for five seconds; then center. Exhale, inhale, and repeat to the left.

7. Place your hands behind your head. Inhale and hyperextend (arch) your lower back. Hold for five seconds, stretching your lower back; then exhale and contract. Use your feet against the wall or sides as a stabilizing force during this movement. Repeat several times.

8. Place your arms alongside your body. Curve your right shoulder toward your right hip, forming a C with your torso, to stretch your left side. Hold for a count of five, and repeat to the other side.

9. Keeping your head and arms relaxed on the bottom of the tub, bend your knees and place your feet flat on the bottom. Bend both knees to the right side to form a spinal twist. Hold for a count of five, then return to center. Repeat to the left side. (You will need to adjust this movement depending on the size of your tub.)

10. Come up onto your side; then sit with your legs straight in front of you. Keep your chin up and your lower back slightly arched as you stretch forward. Grasp the outside of your calves, with your elbows bent and your thumbs on

top. Hold for a count of ten; then release and straighten up.

11. Slide back down to the original position (head on the bottom of the tub and feet elevated). This is a good time for a Healing Moment or your own personal form of prayer. Then visualize your ideal Holistic Triangle and what you are going to do to work toward your goal today. Picture how you'll nourish each side of your Triangle today.

12. Sit up gently, and kneel in the tub. Lather up your body with a fragrant natural soap, and rinse off. Shampoo your hair, if you wish, and lie back to rinse. (If you don't want wet hair, you can use a well-fitting bathing cap during the entire Bathing Ritual.)

13. Let the soapy water out of the tub. Stand up, and use the shower to rinse off with warm water.

14. Slowly adjust the faucets to change the temperature to cold water. At first this may be a shock, but after you're accustomed to the Bathing Ritual, you'll enjoy the cold. Stretch up to the ceiling a few times during this invigorating cold interlude.

15. Finish off with a rinse of warm, but not hot, water.

16. After you get out of the tub and dry off, massage yourself with moisturizer containing natural oils and vitamin E.

On days when you have extra time, you can perform the Bathing Ritual at night as well as in the morning. You can use incense, candlelight, scented bath oils, and music to make it even more sensual.

Although the Bathing Ritual is very pleasurable, remember it's not just a perk that can be sacrificed when you're busy: It has a therapeutic physiological effect. The hot water relaxes your muscles and allows dilation and expansion; the cold water causes contraction, and the warm water brings blood back to your muscles. The exercises are basic stretches to prepare you for the demands of the day. You may hear little cracks and crunches when you perform them; this is the sound of your body adjusting itself.

When you have the time and inclination, you can leave out the shower and perform the entire sequence in the bathtub, filling it up with hot water, then cold water, then warm water. This is also the way to do it if you have a tub but no shower.

If you do not have a bathtub, there is, unfortunately, no way to get the full benefit of weightlessness. To compensate, you can perform the exercises, both physical and mental/spiritual steps, on your exercise mat, then take a hot-cold-warm shower.

HOLISTIC HEALING THERAPIES

Acupressure refers to massage techniques that use manual pressure to stimulate energy points, based on the principles of acupuncture. The pressure serves to stimulate the body's recuperative powers by releasing and balancing the flow of chi.

Chi, which is called prana in India and ki in Japan, is considered the life force or inherent energy within each person. Chi flows through meridians, or energy pathways, and acupressure works to open and balance these meridians. Shiatsu, Jin Shin, do-in, and acu-yoga are some of the forms of acupressure.

Acupuncture involves stimulating the energy points through the insertion of fine needles, the application of heat produced by burning an herb, manual pressure, or a weak electrical current. As in acupressure, the goal is to facilitate the balanced flow of chi throughout the meridians.

The Alexander technique is a method of reducing physical and mental tension by improving habits of posture, balance, coordination, and movement. Alexander teachers offer hands-on guidance and verbal instruction to help their students relearn their innately healthy postures and ways of movement.

Aromatherapy uses aromatic essences extracted from plants. These essential oils are administered by massage, in baths, through skin preparations, compresses, and steam inhalation. Aromatherapists use particular oils for specific conditions, as well as for general beauty treatments and relaxation.

Ayurvedic medicine is the traditional system of healing in India. It is a complex holistic system that incorporates medicinal, psychological, and spiritual principles. Pulse diagnosis, energy points, herbal remedies, dietary counseling, and yoga are some of the modalities utilized in this comprehensive health care system.

Bach Flower Remedies are an outgrowth of homeopathy. Practitioners believe certain plants contain essences that can help reunite the body and soul, nature and spirit. Flower essences are used to strengthen the individual's innate healing power.

Biofeedback training is a technique for learning relaxation and control over automatic body functions. Clients monitor their metabolic changes with the biofeedback machine and learn to evoke relaxation using various techniques.

Body-oriented psychotherapies combine "talk therapy" with body work or movement techniques. Dance movement therapy, for example, uses expressive movement as a therapeutic tool. Bioenergetics, based on the work of Wilhelm Reich, explores the healing power of the body's sexual energy. These and other body-oriented psychotherapies help patients break through psychological barriers that are causing physical symptoms.

Chinese medicine is an ancient holistic system that continues to astound the Western world with its wisdom. Acupuncture, herbal medicine, moxibustion (heat therapy), massage, nutritional advice, and lifestyle counseling are among the techniques used by Chinese doctors.

Chiropractic is now the number one natural health care system in the Western world. As discussed in Chapter 1, traditional chiropractic is based on the principle that the basis of health is an optimally functioning nervous system. The nerve pathways can function properly only when the vertebral bones of the spinal cord are aligned. Misalignment of the vertebrae, called subluxation, puts pressure on the nerves, which can lead to pain, restricted blood supply, and susceptibility to disease. Modern chiropractic is based on the principle that disease is caused by a lack of innate nerve energy with or without subluxation.

"Straight" chiropractors work primarily on realigning the vertebrae through hands-on manipulation and adjustment. Holistic chiropractors utilize additional modalities, which may include massage, physical therapies, rehabilitative exercises, and nutritional counseling. Many of today's chiropractors are holistic physicians who give special attention to the nervous system, musculoskeletal system, spinal biomechanics, and nutrition.

Colonic hydrotherapy is the irrigation of the large intestine through a full enema to cleanse and detoxify. Fasting, saunas and hot tubs, deep breathing, and massage are sometimes used in conjunction with colonic therapy.

Deep tissue body work therapies release and "unstick" the body's connective tissues and muscles to allow them to function properly. The emotional component of posture, breathing, and physical conditions is addressed in some types of deep-tissue body work, such as Rolfing and Hellerwork.

The Feldenkrais method teaches awareness of the skeleton and its muscles and healthier ways to use the body. Teachers use movement training, gentle touch, and verbal dialogue to help students liberate their bodies and relearn the freer movements they had as children.

Herbal medicine, which uses plants in many forms, has been employed in every culture since ancient times to cleanse, heal, and nourish. Herbal medicines trigger biochemical responses in the body and can stimulate the natural healing response. Herbs are used for elimination and detoxification, prevention and health maintenance, toning the organs, nourishing the tissues and blood, and specific healing purposes.

In addition to herbalists, who specialize in prescribing herbal medicine, herbs are used by holistic chiropractors, naturopaths, nutritionists, traditional Chinese doctors, and many other natural healers.

Homeopathy is a system of medicine using preparations of natural essences. It is used for chronic problems, infections, physiological deficiencies, and preventive purposes. Classical homeopaths use homeopathy exclusively, while eclectic homeopaths may use other healing arts, such as vitamin therapy, nutrition, and massage.

Kinesiology is a diagnostic and therapeutic system that employs individual testing of muscles to learn about the patient's overall health. Nutritional counseling, manipulation and pressure point work, and exercise are often used as part of a treatment plan by kinesiologists.

Massage therapy is a system of kneading, stroking, and applying pressure to the body to promote healing, relaxation, cleansing, and general health. One of the most popular forms of massage is Swedish, which uses a series of kneading, friction, and stroking movements over the entire body. Swedish massage improves circulation and releases endorphins, among other effects.

Sports massage focuses on specific muscles and sports injuries. Many massage therapists learn a number of techniques and synthesize their own styles.

Naturopathy is a holistic system of health care based on the belief in the healing power of nature. Naturopaths, or naturopathic physicians, address the underlying cause of disease and use natural means to help restore the body to equilibrium. Herbal remedies, therapeutic diets, supplementation, homeopathic remedies, hydrotherapy, exercise, massage, manipulation, and relaxation training may be included in their practices.

Nutrition therapies use dietary changes and vitamins, minerals, and herbs to heal, promote health, and build immunity. There is a wide variety of nutritional therapies with different philosophies, including macrobiotics, clinical ecologists, and such programs as Pritikin and Atkins.

Physical therapy utilizes massage, exercise, electrical stimulation, ultrasound, and therapeutic exercise to help assist patients recover from disabling conditions and injuries. Physical therapy techniques are also employed by many holistic chiropractors.

Reflexology is a technique in which manual pressure is applied to one part of the body to promote healing in another area and stimulate the innate healing force. Reflexology traces its roots back to the Chinese theory of energy meridians and works to loosen tension and unblock energy flow. It is usually performed on the feet or hands, sometimes in combination with massage.

SELF-MASSAGE

Self-massage is another variation on the age-old healing art of the laying on of hands. While self-massage isn't as sybaritic or therapeutic as receiving a massage, it does have its advantages. It's free of charge and readily available and is a positive way to show your body love and acceptance. Self-massage can also help you become more skilled at massaging other people.

The face, neck, and shoulders are the areas most conducive to self-massage. When you massage your face, be sure it's well lubricated with a natural lotion and the skin is not dry. Keep your nails clipped, and use the flat part of your fingers.

Here is a self-massage sequence for the shoulders, neck, and face.

1. Dim the lights, and lie down on your exercise mat. Begin deep breathing. Let your body sink into the ground, and relax. Let your head feel very heavy and relaxed, your neck elongated.

2. Place your right hand on your left shoulder. Stroke across your left shoulder and up the side of your neck; then up and down behind your ear. Stroke back down to your shoulder. Knead the muscle of your shoulder between your fingers. Do this sequence three times on the left; then use your left hand to massage your right shoulder and the right side of your neck.

3. Place your right thumb in the hollow under your left collarbone and your other fingers under your armpit. Press into the hollow with your thumb in a circular movement. This is a center of lymph nodes and may feel sensitive. Use your left hand on your right side to massage the same area.

4. Relax your head and lengthen your neck. Using both hands, stroke up and down the sides of your neck. Lace your fingers behind your head, and lift your neck into a gentle arch. Hold for fifteen seconds, breathing deeply; then release.

5. Use your thumbs to find sensitive points on your skull.

These points are often at the base of the skull and top of the neck. When you find such a point, press into it with your thumb for ten seconds; then release. You can also massage these spots with a circular motion.

6. Place your fingertips in the center of your forehead. Slowly stroke down your forehead, down your nose, over your cheekbones, then up your temples and across your forehead. Complete five double circles with a slow, gentle movement.

7. Return to any spots that felt tense during the face circles, and massage these areas with minicircles or steady finger pressure.

8. Using all your fingertips, briskly massage your entire scalp with circular movements.

Although an upper body self-massage is most relaxing in a lying-down position, you can also use it as a quick pick-me-up when sitting at work.

1. Tilt your head to one side, and use the opposite hand to stroke up and down your shoulder and the side of your neck. Repeat on the other side.

2. Squeeze the muscles of your shoulders to relieve tightness.

3. Lace your fingers behind your neck, and use them as a cradle as you arch your head up.

To massage your legs, sit with them extended, and knead the muscles with your fingertips. To massage your arms, simply use the opposite hand. Always stroke your limbs toward your heart.

To massage your lower back, either stand or lie on your stomach and rub in a circular motion on the sides of the vertebrae. To relieve sciatic pain, you can massage your buttocks while standing or lying on your stomach.

To massage your own feet, sit in a chair and place one foot on the opposite thigh. Consult a book on reflexology if you want to learn which parts of the foot correspond to different areas of the body and internal organs.

Self-massage can be used as an adjunct to stretching or yoga exercises. As you stretch, you can massage different parts of your body to help them lengthen and relax. Experiment to find out what feels right for you.

HOT AND COLD COMPRESS THERAPY

You'll need two reusable hot and cold packs to use for your self-treatment of muscle pain. Remember, *never put a pack directly on your skin;* always use a towel underneath. Never massage the skin directly after using hot or cold packs; wait until it has returned to normal temperature. People with skin conditions, children, and elderly people should be particularly careful about compresses and seek the advice of a health professional before using them.

1. Place a towel warmed with hot water on the muscle or area where you are experiencing the most tension or pain. Then place the hot pack on the towel for fifteen to twenty minutes. This allows the muscle to relax and expand and increases blood circulation to the area.
2. Remove the hot pack and warm towel. Wait a few minutes for skin temperature to return to normal. Then place a cold, wet towel and an ice pack on the area. You can compress the muscle by lying on the pack if you wish. Be aware the cold may be uncomfortable and you may experience burning, pain, and numbness. Use the cold pack for no longer than ten minutes. The cold works by constricting the muscle, which removes the old blood and metabolic wastes.
3. Wait until the skin is normal temperature. Again, place a warm towel and a hot pack on the area for fifteen to twenty minutes. This allows the muscle to expand and fresh, oxygenated blood to enter.

Remove the hot pack and relax for a few minutes. Mentally send the muscle your healing energy. Rise gently, and avoid using the muscle strenuously for the next hour.

Bibliography/
Suggested Further Reading

HOLISTIC HEALTH

Bliss, Shepherd, ed. *The New Holistic Health Handbook.* Lexington, Mass.: Stephen Greene Press, 1985.

Melville, Arabella, and Colin Johnson. *Health Without Drugs: Alternatives to Prescriptions and Over-the-Counter Medicines.* New York: Simon & Schuster, 1990.

Mendelsohn, Robert S. *Confessions of a Medical Heretic.* Chicago: Contemporary Books, 1979.

Olsen, Kristin Gottschalk. *The Encyclopedia of Alternative Health Care.* New York: Simon & Schuster, 1990.

Pilkington, J. Maya, and the Diagram Group. *Alternative Healing and Your Health.* New York: Ballantine Books, 1991.

MENTAL/SPIRITUAL SIDE

Benson, Herbert, and Miriam Z. Klipper. *The Relaxation Response.* New York: Avon, 1976.

Borysenko, Joan, with Larry Rothstein. *Minding the Body, Mending the Mind.* New York: Bantam Books, 1988.

Chopra, Deepak. *Quantum Healing: Exploring the Frontiers of The Mind/Body Medicine.* New York: Bantam Books, 1989.

Gawain, Shakti. *Creative Visualization.* New York: Bantam, 1982.

Hay, Louise L. *You Can Heal Your Life.* Santa Monica, Calif.: Hay House, 1984.

LeShan, Lawrence. *How to Meditate.* New York: Bantam Books, 1974.

Miller, Ronald S. *As Above, So Below: Paths to Spiritual Renewal in Daily Life.* Los Angeles: Jeremy P. Tarcher, 1992.

Padmus, Emrika, and the Editors of *Prevention* Magazine. *The Complete Guide to Your Emotions and Your Health.* Emmaus, Pa.: Rodale Press, 1986.

Thich Nhat Han. *The Miracle of Mindfulness.* Boston: Beacon Press, 1987.

CHEMICAL SIDE

Airola, Paavo. *Hypoglycemia: A Better Approach.* Sherwood, Ore.: Health Plus, 1977.

Balch, James F. and Phyllis A. *Prescription for Nutritional Healing.* Garden City Park, N.Y.: Avery Publishing, 1990.

Blauer, Stephen. *Juicing for Life.* Garden City Park, N.Y.: Avery Publishing, 1989.

Buchman, Dian Dincin. *Herbal Medicine.* New York: Gramercy, 1980.

Diamond, Harvey and Marilyn. *Fit for Life II: Living Health.* New York: Warner Books, 1987.

Dunne, Lavon J. *Nutrition Almanac.* New York: McGraw-Hill, 1975.

Gershoff, Stanley, with Catherine Whitney. *The Tufts University Guide to Total Nutrition.* New York: HarperCollins, 1991.

Graedon, Joe. *The New People's Pharmacy.* New York: Bantam, 1985.

Long, James W. *Essential Guide to Prescription Drugs.* New York: HarperCollins, 1993.

Kloss, Jethro. *Back to Eden.* Loma Linda, Calif.: Back to Eden Publishing, 1939.

McDougall, John A. and Mary A. *The McDougall Plan.* Clinton, N.J.: New Win Publishing, 1983.

Mindell, Earl. *Earl Mindell's Herb Bible.* New York: Simon & Schuster, 1992.

———. *Earl Mindell's Vitamin Bible.* New York: Warner Books, 1979.

Muir, Murray, and Joseph Pizzorno. *Encyclopedia of Natural Medicine.* Rocklin, Calif.: Prima Publishing, 1991.

Murray, Michael T. *The Complete Book of Juicing.* Rocklin, Calif.: Prima Publishing, 1992.

Null, Gary. *Clearer, Cleaner, Safer, Greener: A Blueprint for Detoxifying Your Environment.* New York: Random House, 1990.

———. *No More Allergies.* New York: Villard, 1992.

Robbins, John. *Diet for a New America.* Walpole, N.H.: Stillpoint Publishing, 1987.

———. *May All Be Fed: Diet for a New World.* New York: William Morrow, 1992.

Wade, Carlson. *Immune Power Boosters: Your Key to Feeling Younger, Living Longer.* New York: Prentice Hall, 1990.

PHYSICAL SIDE

Anderson, Bob. *Stretching.* Bolinas, Calif.: Shelter, 1980.

Cooper, Kenneth H. *The Aerobics Program for Total Well-Being: Exercise, Diet, Emotional Balance.* New York: M. Evans, 1982.

Evans, William, and Irwin Rosenberg, with Jacqueline Thompson. *Biomarkers: The 10 Keys to Longevity.* New York: Simon & Schuster, 1992.

Glover, Bob, and Jack Shepherd. *Runner's Handbook.* New York: Penguin, 1985.

Hittleman, Richard. *Yoga: 28 Day Exercise Plan.* New York: Bantam Books, 1973.

Lidell, Lucinda. *The Book of Massage.* New York: Simon & Schuster, 1984.

Vishnu-devananda, Swami. *The Complete Illustrated Book of Yoga.* New York: Pocket Books, 1981.

FURTHER READING ON MAJOR DISEASES

Bennett, Cleaves M. *Control Your High Blood Pressure Without Drugs.* New York: Doubleday, 1984.

Dreher, Henry. *Your Defense Against Cancer.* New York: Harper & Row, 1989.

Heimlich, Jane. *What Your Doctor Won't Tell You.* New York: HarperCollins, 1990.

Matthews-Simonton, Stephanie, and O. Carl Simonton. *Getting Well Again.* New York: Bantam Books, 1979.

Null, Gary. *Healing Your Body Naturally: Alternative Treatments to Illness.* New York: Four Walls, Eight Windows, 1992.

Ornish, Dean. *Dr. Dean Ornish's Program for Reversing Heart Disease.* New York: Random House, 1990.

Siegel, Bernie S. *Love, Medicine and Miracles.* New York: Harper & Row, 1986.

———. *Peace, Love & Healing.* New York: Harper & Row, 1990.

Whitaker, Julian M. *Reversing Diabetes.* New York: Warner Books, 1990.

———. *Reversing Heart Disease.* New York: Warner Books, 1985.

Index

Entries in **boldface** refer to tables and illustrations.